# Health and Culture

To my late parents

my father, Airhihenbuwa Obadolagbon
my mother, Igbinosa Osomwota
my other father (my wife's father), Jean-Victor Kingué

that we may bear the torch you have passed on to us
with the strength, humility, and wholesomeness
that your lives embodied

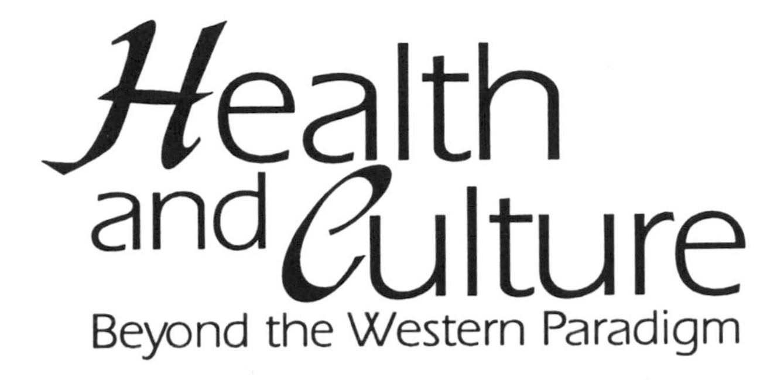


Collins O. Airhihenbuwa

**SAGE** Publications
*International Educational and Professional Publisher*
Thousand Oaks London New Delhi

Cover photograph and chapter opening details by Dave Beese. From the author's personal collection of African art.

*For information address:*

SAGE Publications, Inc.
2455 Teller Road
Thousand Oaks, California 91320

SAGE Publications Ltd.
6 Bonhill Street
London EC2A 4PU
United Kingdom

SAGE Publications India Pvt. Ltd.
M-32 Market
Greater Kailash I
New Delhi 110 048 India

Printed in the United States of America

**Library of Congress Cataloging-in-Publication Data**

Airhihenbuwa, Collins O.
Health and culture: beyond the western paradigm / Collins O. Airhihenbuwa.
p. cm.
Includes bibliographical references and index.
ISBN 0-8039-7156-7 (hbk.: acid-free paper).—ISBN 0-8039-7157-5 (pbk.: acid-free paper)
1. Social medicine—Africa. 2. Health promotion—Social aspects—Africa. 3. Preventive health services—Social aspects—Africa. 4. Ethnocentrism. I. Title.
RA418.3.A35A37 1995
306.4'61'096—dc20 95-2551

This book is printed on acid-free paper.

95 96 97 98 99 10 9 8 7 6 5 4 3 2 1

Sage Production Editor: Diane S. Foster
Sage Typesetter: Andrea D. Swanson

# Contents

# *Acknowledgments*

I pour libation to my ancestors for their spiritual foundations on which the seed of my intellectual curiosity continues to be fertilized and nurtured. My personal and professional growth has been shaped by my Edo cultural values and meanings, on which my humanity is affirmed and legitimated. My humanity continues to be fulfilled by the sense of cultural awareness and pride that were instilled in me by my late mother and father.

A debt of gratitude is owed to many people for their encouragement and support in the completion of this book. First and foremost is my wife, Angèle M. Kingué, for her love and caring and the challenge and inspiration her intellectual, cultural, and moral insights have kindled in me. Next is my son, Iyare, for the reward of being a part of his youthful transformation and the sober reminder that the measure of human progress is a function of how far we have journeyed rather than the time at which we arrive at a destination. I thank also my brother, Osa, for unwavering support in his review of the initial draft of this book, and my dear friend Linden Lewis for his painstaking efforts in providing detailed and insightful feedback on another draft. Linden has been particularly generous with his intellectual richness by providing me with important essays and critiques as well as his brotherly support in nurturing our kindred spirit. I am thankful to Emmanuel Eze for his critique and feedback in the preparation of this book. I also owe a debt of gratitude to my friend and mentor, James B. Stewart, for his towering and unequivocal support over the years. Jim has been a guiding light in providing feedback in the preparation of several of my published works. This book was no exception. His thorough and selfless dedication to excellence provides a model to which I aspire.

Many thanks go to several of my students over the years, from whom I have learned so much. They are too many to identify by name, and yet I feel obliged to name two of them: Leonard Jack, Jr., with whom I have collaborated on several projects and who continues to be a close and valued friend and colleague; and Michael Ludwig, who has deepened my appreciation for dialogic education in more than one way. In preparing this book, I drew on the many writings of outstanding educational theorists and cultural critics. Among them is Henry Giroux, from whom, through personal interaction, I have been fortunate to have gained unparalleled intellectual stimulation. He has been very generous with his time in providing me with valuable feedback on a draft of this book.

Many others have directly and indirectly nourished my scholarly appetite as well as enriched my personal and professional growth. They include Harold Cheatham, Carrie Dickens-Guscott, Shiriki Kumanyika, Cathy Lyons, Richard Smith, and Dory Storms. I am grateful also to my coauthors on previous publications, particularly Ira E. Harrison, Agatha Lowe, Ralph DiClemente, and Gina Wingood.

Portions of this book have appeared elsewhere in different form, and I would like to express my sincere gratitude to my previous publishers for their permission to make use of certain materials. Finally, I would like to thank my editors at Sage Publications, Christine Smedley, Diane Foster, and Judy Selhorst for their support in the final production of this book.

Although the support I have received from others has been extensive across my personal and professional extended family, any mistakes and errors in this book are solely mine.

# *Introduction*

> Where one thing stands, another thing must stand beside it. . . . This saying "there is only one way" is something which is new to my people.
>
> *Chinua Achebe, interview, 1992*

The African philosophy of life invoked by Achebe in the above epigraph is the bedrock upon which the discourse in this book is grounded. This philosophy of the human construction of reality, as lived in many African cultures, underscores an embracing of multiple truths relative to health, education, politics, religion, valuation, and thus decision-making processes. This ideology, which shuns the "all or nothing" mentality of Western culture and its attendant promotion of universal truths, should be understood not only for its counterpoising principle and quality but as a different genre.

In this book I challenge traditional paradigms in health, education, and development on three primary, yet complementary, fronts. The first is the valorization of Eurocentrism and patriarchy in the production and acquisition of health knowledge and health behavior, coupled with the continued oppression and suppression of cultural expressions of non-Western peoples and women. The second principle is the reliance on the notion of "development" as an emancipatory process even though this concept is grounded in the promotion of Western hegemony in the name of universal progress. Development ideology valorizes standardization through the notion of universal truths in the name of a common global mission. The third principle, which relates directly to the first two, is the overemphasis of health promotion and disease prevention practices in the medical model of prevention. Consequently, the health education/promotion discipline has failed to ground its professional (both philosophical and practical) praxis adequately in such areas of humanities as philosophy, history, and cultural studies. The result has been the absence of meaningful participation of people and their cultures in positive behavioral transformation where appropriate. It has become common practice in the field of public health and in the social and behavioral sciences to pay lip service to the importance of culture in the study and understanding of health behaviors, but culture has yet to be inscribed at the root of health promotion and disease prevention programs, at least in any manner that legitimates its centrality in public health praxis.

Health promotion and disease prevention practices continue to operate under the strong and direct influence of the medical Westernized model of prevention. Although benefits are derived from such influence, it seems unconscionable that a profession that anchors its raison d'être in the ability to influence human behavior has consistently undermined and in most cases ignored the centrality of culture (as evident in the mission of cultural studies, for example) in health and education. There continues to be strong reliance on medicine and individual psychology, even though such orientation has constantly been challenged for its limitations, which are driven by monocentrism and often result in cultural inappropriateness. For example, as Chow (1991) notes, psychoanalysis is a Western practice that focuses on the private self, whereas the Chinese and those in many other non-Western cultures are more concerned with public life and the larger issues of history than with privacy. Thus psychoanalysis is culturally inappropriate in many non-Western countries. From this vantage point, health promotion must learn from the problems encountered by Western "development" specialists in attempting to guide societal change in non-Western nations.

The ideology behind the concept of development has reified Western hegemony by anchoring measures of "progress" in the values and principles of the West. "Only from the vantage point of the West is it possible to define the 'third world' as underdeveloped and economically dependent. Without the overdetermined discourse that creates the third world, there would be no (singular and privileged) first world" (Mohanty, 1991b, p. 74). Development conceived of as a prepackaged formula that is manufactured only in Northern nations for application in Southern nations is now an outmoded construct (Sachs, 1992). This concept, with its appropriation of Southern nations as "underdeveloped," was injected into popular discourse on January 20, 1949, by Harry S Truman. After more than 40 years of exposing the historical genealogy of the disempowering and nonparticipatory nature of the concept of development, a new concept—globalization— is now invoked that is equally disempowering, because it promises to marginalize further the cultural expressions of Southern nations. Although globalization—as theorized from political, sociological, economic, environmental, geographic, and even historical perspectives—may have begun as a process of integration and incorporation of national economies into a global one, the appropriation of globalization in the areas of health and human development as "a marker for progress" has become the inevitable outcome.

At the end of the twentieth century, globalization has been introduced into popular discourse as the new language of universal truth. The life support of globalization rests on fulfilling the "needs" of the "wretched of the earth" (Fanon, 1968) and the "faces at the bottom of the well" (Bell, 1992). "Just as 'needs' became an important emblem which allowed managers to provide a philanthropic rationale for the destruction of cultures, so, now, needs are being replaced by the new emblem of 'basic requirements' under which the new goal, 'survival of the earth' can be justified" (Illich, 1992, p. 98). Like its predecessor, development, globalization is acultural and promises further to medicalize and psychologize, in the Western sense, human behavior, such that non-Western cultures are expected to maintain their "underdeveloped" state and play catch-up, as is currently the case in many African countries.

The investigation undertaken in this book is based on the premise that African theory and practice, particularly within the context of health, must be rooted in African cultural codes and meaning. The focus here is not on cultural relativism, but on problematizing the notion of universal truth. In explicating African cultural productions,

"Western interpreters as well as African analysts have been using categories and conceptual systems which depend on a Western epistemological order" (Mudimbe, 1988, p. x). This is particularly salient in the discourse on health and education in Africa. Progressive discourses/theories of today—postmodern, postcolonial, feminist, and cultural studies—have challenged classical paradigms by advocating representation, or what Stuart Hall (1991) calls the "third space." However, these theories/discourses have failed to address health adequately as a cultural production. Whereas the various inputs into cultural production are shaped by elements of the fields of humanity, the output of cultural production is realized in the health status of individuals and the health conditions of societies.

To invoke the centrality of culture in public health and health promotion activities is to challenge health promotion and disease prevention approaches that overlook or downplay the importance of history, politics, and education in shaping the landscape of cultural production. Further, it is to deepen and extend the possibilities of progressive approaches, such as critical pedagogy and cultural studies, that centralize culture in their theories and practices. The accomplishment of these tasks requires the deconstruction of existing systems of dominant values in a manner that challenges the very foundation of the social and cultural order. Such a challenge is not merely to destroy a few prejudices; rather, it is to see through the revolving door of all rationalizations by meeting head-on the truth of the struggle between fiction and reality (Minh-ha, 1991). The centrality of culture in health and education initiatives is a discourse that resonates with the politics of representation, which are affirmed through voices of various cultural expressions and meanings. Cultural workers who are engaged in the politics of representation seek to deconstruct (analyze the historical genealogy of) the anthropologization of meaning in many health promotion and disease prevention programs. Stated differently, the terrain of health promotion programs is replete with pejorative cultural codes and meanings anchored in Eurocentric and Westernized ideology. The tension that results is manifested in the practices of behavioral and social scientists, such as anthropologists (even those with the best of intentions), whose actions, by the nature of their professional episteme, imply the silence of "Others." An unresolvable problem of anthropology is essentially that it is a discourse of representation of Others who are defined epistemologically as inferior, silent, and in need of being spoken for (Said, in Mariani & Crary, 1990). In the words of Trinh T. Minh-ha (1989), anthropology is "mainly a conversation of 'us' with 'us' about 'them,' of the white man with the white man about the primitive-nature man . . . in which 'them' is silent" (pp. 65-67; quoted in Alcoff, 1991-1992, p. 6).

In the United States, the appropriation of jazz by external interests and its translation into symbolic representations that allow mimicry is an example of how anthropologizing is operationalized within a culture and can manipulate the cultural rules in ways not conceivable by indigenous members (Stewart, 1992). Although the concern about speaking for others has always been focused on anthropologists, the fact remains that many behavioral and social scientists, including public health and health education professionals, engage in anthropologization of meaning. In their desire to raise levels of awareness about non-Western cultures, these professionals ground their theories and practices in a Westernized gaze. By so doing, they often obscure and distort the meanings, and thus the reporting, of what they observe. When this occurs, even though it may be inadvertent, the outcome is misrepresentation of the cultural codes and meanings of non-Western cultures. Such misrepresentation dehistoricizes cultural codes and meanings and truncates their cultural genealogy and transformative possibilities. What often results is the periodization of cultural practices as archival remains, invoking a notion that the present has no link to the past, and thus erasing historical continuity. Yet the most efficient cultural weapon with which a people can arm itself is the feeling of historical continuity (Diop, 1981).

Cultures and traditions are simply the forms of social interaction accepted by particular communities at particular times, and according to their worldviews and historical experiences, such that there are several alternatives and systems of values selected for their usefulness (Akinjogbin, 1987/1990). In other words, contrary to popular notions, culture is *not* past values and practices that have fossilized at a particular point in history, never to change and recounted only orally in the present. Values and practices that remain in the past and are no longer practiced should not be considered (for all practical purposes) part of an active culture and tradition. The notion that culture and tradition are practices engaged in the past and therefore should be forgotten only promotes cultural amnesia. And as Chinweizu (1987) has noted, those who would teach us amnesia about our past, especially while doping us with accounts of the pasts of other peoples, cannot have our best interests at heart. They wish us to commit social and cultural suicide by turning into zombies.

Cultures are not static. They change over time in accordance with the interpretive values, beliefs, norms, and practices of the group, whose members define and live by the ideals of those practices and values. Very often culture is blamed for certain ill-understood health practices, when in fact the culprit is the lofty interpretation of culture for the maintenance of imperial dominance and hegemony. This has been particularly true when Westernized professionals have addressed issues of health beliefs and practices in African societies.

Preventive health programs that are anchored in culturally appropriate paradigms enhance and magnify the possibilities offered in progressive educational processes/approaches that embrace dialogic participation. This process of engaging teachers/interventionists and students/audiences in the production of meaning, value, pleasure, and knowledge should be central to the mission of health promotion and education. It is only through such dialogue that varied cultural expressions and meanings are affirmed and centralized, and the production of cultural identity can be legitimating and empowering relative to promoting individual, family, community, and societal health.

This book is presented in two parts. Part I addresses the theoretical and philosophical grounding of the reciprocity between health and culture within the African context. Chapter 1 offers a discussion of health promotion and the discourse on culture and development. Chapter 2 then magnifies the salience of the theme presented in Chapter 1 by focusing on the importance of cultural codes in health communication. In Chapter 3, I introduce a cultural model (PEN-3) for decolonizing health and education programs, linking theory with practice in the development of health promotion and disease prevention programs. This programmatic method offers researchers and practitioners the opportunity to understand and evaluate culture from multiple dimensions, instead of appropriating culture only as a barrier.

The five chapters in Part II offer theoretical and practical insights into the politics of representation in the discourse on health promotion and present examples of the application of the PEN-3 model for specific populations and traditional healing modalities. In Chapter 4, the historical and cultural context of traditional medicine is presented, with examples of how this modality can be strengthened from within its cultural space to maximize its benefit for global health. Chapter 5 addresses women's health issues as a construct of patriarchal hegemony on the one hand and Westernized female hegemony on the other. The discussion focuses on the degree to which these combined forces negate the voices of African women and thus compromise their health status and the information available to them about their health concerns, such as menopause. Chapter 6 examines the health concerns of children and youth and the sociocultural production of youth within the African context. Data are presented on the health conditions of children and youth to underscore the way in which the silencing of youth by adults has contributed to children's poor health conditions. Chapter 7 addresses the health concerns of African Americans within the context of culture. Identity formation relative to the politics of representation is presented as a backdrop for a discussion of how culture mediates and is mediated by individual, family, and society. Thus the challenge of individual possibilities against the weight of societal constraint is discussed within the context of empowerment. The mythology of health care as a "delivery system" is problematized through a focus on the way in which the system renders selective services that are dictated through the power of medical production. Chapter 8 presents a futuristic approach to health promotion as a challenge to move beyond the decolonization of health and education as a cultural, political, and educational project. Such a challenge requires that the fields of health and education draw from the theories and practices of cultural studies and other areas of the humanities rather than rely solely on the medical model in addressing health problems in Africa.

Although the totalizing of African experiences does not always accurately reflect Africa's intraregional diversity, it is often invoked, mostly because of shared colonial and postcolonial experiences and political and economic oppression that continues to be inscribed in the policies of international agencies such as the International Monetary

Fund, the World Bank, and the World Health Organization. This book invites scholars and cultural workers committed to the politics of representation in health, education, and development to engage in a "polylogue" designed to create a space in which voices of various intellectual and programmatic discourses are affirmed and legitimated. The discussion that follows recognizes and inscribes culture at the core of understanding and influencing health behavior in a manner that centers the oppressed and marginalized in creating and managing their collective destinies. Such a transformative process reinforces Chinua Achebe's words of wisdom, which have been echoed by Chinweizu, reminding us that the West has not put the final touches on creation, because it is morning yet on creation day.

# PART I

# THEORIZING HEALTH AND CULTURE IN THE AFRICAN CONTEXT

# 1

# Culture, Health Promotion, and Development

> To a large extent culture and health coincide. Each culture gives shape to a unique *Gestalt* of health and to a unique conformation of attitudes towards pain, disease, impairment, and death, each of which designates a class of that human performance that has traditionally been called the art of suffering.
>
> *Ivan Illich,* Medical Nemesis, *1976*

> The point about our development is not the supervisory transfer to us of their expertise, but our development of our own. And the way to develop Nigerian expertise is by giving ourselves the opportunity to try, fail, learn and succeed.
>
> *Chinweizu,* Decolonizing the African Mind, *1987*

Culture is a system of interrelated values active enough to influence and condition perception, judgment, communication, and behavior in a given society (Mazrui, 1986, p. 239). Culture is as much a structure as it is economic and political, and it is rooted in institutions such as families and schools as well as in communications industries (West, 1993). When addressing the issues of identity and difference within the contexts of power, agency, and history, we must foreground the political dimensions of culture in the process of transformation (Giroux, 1994b). Culture must be understood within the context of its transformative possibilities rather than according to the unilineal measure of the West that has come to be known as *development.*

The concept of development—or its ideological appropriation for Southern nations, *underdevelopment*—has been used by scholars from both Northern and Southern nations as a marker for what is considered to be an acceptable economic threshold that Southern nations must exceed in order to experience "progress." Since 1949, when Harry S Truman introduced the phrase "underdeveloped countries" into popular discourse, the hidden agenda for development has been nothing less than the Westernization of the world (for detailed discussion of this point, see Sachs, 1992). This process has entered a new discourse at the end of the twentieth century with the valorization of *globalization.* Globalization, as a concept produced within the context of global changes, has tended to focus only on economic production, capital restructuring, and their attendant political implications, with little regard for negative cultural changes in global societies. Globalization, within health and human development constructs—like its predecessor, development—promises an acultural world, where an individual can be at home anywhere. Development concepts inherited missionary ideology: crusading to redeem converts and to "help" them get to the threshold of "progress" as defined by the West (Gronemeyer, 1992).

Unfortunately, for people in Southern nations, who make up two-thirds of the world's population, development efforts resonate with perceptions of themselves as underdeveloped, with all the pejorative connotations that it carries (Esteva, 1992). For many African countries, *development* and *progress* have come to mean growth in gross national product, even though such an equation has been long rejected by those who initiated and promoted it, including the World Bank. African development is not merely a matter of growth in GNP statistics; it is a matter of shaping certain cultural institutions, of creating and elevating critical consciousness in the African population, so that this consciousness can properly guide the production, distribution, and consumption of the items usually reflected in GNP figures (Chinweizu, Jemie, & Madubuike, 1983). The myriad positive and progressive values and mores that enabled African countries to withstand the emotional, psychological, and physical violence of colonial as well as postcolonial oppression are being forsaken for what is believed to be the path to progress. Progress is now believed to be a natural outgrowth of development, which in turn is believed to be concomitant with modernization. Modernization and development are touted as the twin engines of progress, even though the economic policies advanced by modernization have been incapable of addressing the transformation of the productive forces and productive relations that lead to progress. Modernization has been nothing more than an attempt at Westernization and ideological containment of Southern nations in the name of development. Freire (1973) has observed that although development may mean modernization, not all modernization leads to development. For example, nuclear waste dumping and infant formula production continue to lead to increased morbidity and mortality, resulting in societal regression in conditions of living. This reality has become increasingly evident in assessments of the impacts and outcomes of numerous health and education programs planned for and implemented in Southern nations.

At the center of health and education initiatives is the ability to look to our past, not only for historical continuity but for understanding about the trials, failures, and possibilities that shape our individual and collective experiences. "We affirm the ties of the past, the bonds of the present, when we relearn our history, nurture the shared sensibility that has been retained in the present, linking these gestures to resistance struggle, to liberation movements that seek to eradicate domination and transform society" (hooks, 1992, p. 194). As Stuart Hall (1991) notes, the relation that peoples of the world have to their own past is a part of the discovery and affirmation of their own ethnicity: "The past is not only a position from which to speak, but it is also an absolutely necessary resource in what one has to say" (p. 18). These past and present experiences constitute a group's cultural identity.

Cultural identity is based primarily on shared historical, linguistic, and psychological lineage (Diop, 1991). These sets of collective factors in a culture influence the group's design for living, the shared set of socially transmitted perceptions about the nature of the physical, social, and spiritual world, particularly as it relates to achieving life's goals (Basch, 1990). As Henry Giroux (1992) observes, culture "is not an object of unquestioning reverence but a mobile field of ideological and material relations that are unfinished, multilayered, and always open to interrogation" (p. 99). "Culture embodies those moral, ethical and aesthetic values, the set of spiritual eyeglasses, through which people come to view themselves and their place in the universe. Language as a culture is the collective memory bank of a people's experience in history" (Thiong'O, 1993, p. 14). Those who develop health and education programs must examine carefully the differences as well as the similarities in cultural perceptions, so as to understand health beliefs and practices more fully and to address them appropriately within their particular contexts. Such understanding should not be based on market economy and buying power, the traditional indices of development. Culture develops within the process of a people wrestling with the natural and social environment, and thus embodies the moral, aesthetic, and ethical values that are manifested in the people's consciousness (Thiong'O, 1993).

Important aspects of cultural expression in African countries are found in aesthetic values and meanings as evident in arts, music, and clothing. Such values and meanings are laden with desires, emotions, and expectations that may not be discernible through Westernized code. For example, "the notion of religion is hardly ever used [by Westerners] to designate African beliefs and religious practices" (Mudimbe, 1988, p. 76). In an attempt to show "the ways things really are" in the non-West, we have become engaged in discourses that produce a non-West that is deprived of fantasy, desires, and contradictory emotions (Chow, 1991). It is the omission of these aesthetic values from the analytic framework used to examine African cultures that renders external approaches to African experience Eurocentric. Marxist literary criticism is limited by its insistence on the tendency to base aesthetic assessment solely on how the market economy shapes the political struggle of the proletariat. This market-driven analysis tends to make Marxist literary criticism thin on what are commonly considered aesthetic concerns in African traditions, thus ignoring, or denouncing as "formalism," questions of beauty, style, technique, sensibility, and appropriateness, which are at the core of African aesthetics (Chinweizu, 1987).

In health promotion and behavior change programs, *cultural sensitivity* refers to the need to develop programs in ways that are consistent with a people's and community's cultural framework, rather than based on the Western paradigm within which most health, education, and development programs are planned, implemented, and evaluated. Health denotes a process of adaptation. It is the result not of instinct, but of an autonomous yet culturally shaped reaction to socially created reality (Illich, 1976). For example, illness is a socially recognized state, carrying with it certain specific drawbacks, obligations, and privileges, depending on the circumstances (Basch, 1990). Each culture creates its own responses to health and disease. For the same symptoms—of kleptomania, for example—in different cultures, an individual might be executed, sentenced to death, exiled, hospitalized, or given arms or tax money (Illich, 1976).

## The Discourse of Difference in Health and Education

Eurocentric approaches to global educational processes should be deconstructed and reconstructed to reflect varied cultural expressions. Attempts to affirm cultural differences in schools and communities often manifest themselves in calls for program and curriculum integration, although program/curriculum reformation/transformation is a more progressive approach to centralizing diversity in the learning process. In some cases, special programs are developed to redress the grievances of the marginalized. Racism is often atoned for through measures aimed at eliminating racist institutional barriers in the marketplace and through the provision of compensatory programs to enhance the cultural capital and skills of the oppressed, as has been evident in various remedial programs designed for African Americans in schools and the workplace (Giroux, 1992).

In a culture-centered approach to health and education, the experiences of the Others must be centralized in the mainstream school curriculum for the benefit of students from both the center and the margin. "To open up to the culture's soul is to allow one to become wet, to become soaked in the cultural and historical waters of those individuals who are involved in the experience" (Freire, 1993, p. 106). Such involvement and total commitment are transformative for both the interventionists and the target population. The resulting reformation of the curriculum/programmatic paradigm includes affirmation and encouragement of different languages of expression, health beliefs, and cultural values. For example, binary opposition is unnecessarily constructed between modern information channels that are based on the Western construct and traditional information channels (oral communication). Both systems of communication are effectively functional within their contexts; in some cases, the two are quite complementary. Unfortunately, many health communication programs in the past have negated a form of cultural production by ignoring oral communication. This has been true particularly in the planning, implementation, and evaluation of programs in many African cultures. Ngugi Wa Thiong'O (1993) notes that the biggest weapon wielded and unleashed daily by imperialism against the oppressed and the exploited of the earth is the cultural bomb:

> The effect of a cultural bomb is to annihilate a people's belief in their names, in their languages, in their environment, in their heritage of struggle, in their unity, in their capacities and ultimately in themselves. It makes them see their past as one wasteland of non-achievement and it makes them want to distance themselves from the wasteland. (p. 3)

Ultimately, a broader discourse on the politics of representation in health promotion calls for the decolonization of the minds of the members of the marginalized group. Africans, Asians, Latin Americans, as well as African Americans and members of other U.S. minority groups, must insist on appropriate representation in the production of knowledge and cultural identity, particularly concerning learning opportunities in health and development. Although some interventionists understand and respect the value of oral tradition, the programmatic response to this form of cultural expression tends to focus only on the storyteller. This is consistent with classical pedagogy, which positions the teacher/educator as the ultimate repository of knowledge and relegates students to the status of objects that cannot produce knowledge but can only acquire it. Ultimately, the teacher/educator is disempowered by the failure to engage the learner in the production of knowledge such that the terrain of learning is multiaccented and mutually enriching. In an attempt to construct what they believe to be a terrain of learning for the voiceless, interventionists assume the role of the storyteller by constructing stories under the guise of cultural sensitivity. Such an approach fails to understand the dynamic of the story listener, which is as equally important as, if not more important than, that of the storyteller.

Cultural dynamics such as communication codes, meanings, and context between the storyteller and listener promote knowledge production and acquisition. Thus oral tradition generally is not only the heritage of the spoken or sung word; it is also the heritage of the ear (Faseke, 1990). Stated differently, people in oral traditional cultures (as in many African countries) are accustomed to learning by listening. Learning by seeing is important to the extent that what is seen is congruent with what is heard. Critical aspects of learning by listening include *who* was speaking, the way the words were said, and in what context. This issue raises questions about the ethical and cultural incongruence of assuming the role of storyteller without training or education for that role, and without a thorough understanding of the cultural implications of storytelling for learning. I do not mean to generalize here about all African cultures as cultures of the ear; rather, I want to emphasize the importance of taking this form of cultural expression into account in health intervention projects as a valued form and sometimes the primary form of cultural production. Storytelling requires that one immerse oneself in the storytelling tradition, undergo appropriate apprenticeship, master the verbal arts, and be able to write one's own re-creations of traditional stories (Chinweizu et al., 1983). The storyteller, through whom truth is summoned to unwind itself to the audience, is a creator, a delighter, and a teacher (Minh-ha, 1991).

Given the realities of cultural production, we can conclude that the use of posters, flyers, and other pictorial learning tools in health promotion and health communication programs may have limited, if any, impacts in many cultures. Even when such materials are culturally appropriate, there are still questions to be addressed with respect to when and how they should be used. Alternative methods of cross-cultural communication should be explored to ensure that the process does not disempower the target group. When listening is the culturally appropriate method of learning, health professionals involved in developing, implementing, and evaluating programs in cultures other than their own should be required to develop the requisite skills for effective and meaningful program implementation. Furthermore, institutions of higher learning that have claimed intellectual hegemony over teaching and learning should reform their health curricula to reflect the cultural realities of the global population. Chapter 2 addresses the role of culture in communication, particularly as it relates to health information and beliefs.

# 2

# Communicating Health Within Culture

> I do not believe that the mass-media change people's attitudes and beliefs, but I believe that LEARNING EXPERIENCES do. The mass-media are influential in so far as they are, or can be, part of good learning experiences.
>
> *Andreas Fuglesang*, Applied Communication in Developing Countries, *1973*

Cultural codes, symbols, and values embody the essence of meaning that people bring to the production and acquisition of knowledge. These forms of cultural expression are accented in the meanings that participants bring to the communication of health messages. The dialogic process necessarily accents verbal and nonverbal exchange such that participants' behaviors are culturally meaningful.

Health educators and those who design health promotion and disease prevention programs must examine health behaviors in particular cultures in terms of whether or not they are rooted in the cultural values and beliefs of the people. For example, it has been demonstrated that in several African countries, person-to-person

---

AUTHOR'S NOTE: This chapter contains a brief portion of my article "Health Promotion and the Discourse on Culture: Implications for Empowerment," *Health Education Quarterly, 21*(3), 345-353. Copyright © 1994 by John Wiley & Sons, Inc., Publishers. Reprinted by permission.

communication (through home visits) has been more effective in changing negative health behaviors than have messages distributed through the mass media. This finding is undoubtedly related to the oral tradition that is the customary bedrock for the production and acquisition of knowledge, as well as the construction of reality, in African cultures. Educating students and audiences serves as an introduction to how a culture is organized, a demonstration of who should speak for whom, and what within the culture is considered invalid and unworthy of public recognition (Giroux, 1992).

## Health Promotion and Cultural Communication

If the bullet is the means of physical subjugation, language is the means of spiritual subjugation (Thiong'O, 1986). Fuglesang (1973) concludes that the most effective method of learning is through demonstration, because the learner uses all the senses—hearing, smell, vision, taste, and touch. Unfortunately, most of the health communication programs that have been implemented in Southern nations have emphasized only visual learning. Fuglesang also notes that visual literacy is an acquired skill.

Central to the issue of cultural variance in the production and acquisition of knowledge (as discussed in Chapter 1) is how the notion of visual literacy as a "superior form of learning" devalues orature and orality, as theorized and practiced in many African countries, as forms of cultural production. Seeing and/or visualizing, as expressed in such idioms as "You see what I mean" and "Get the picture?" are more symbolic of mental imagery than of visual learning, although visualizing can serve as reinforcer. The notion of knowledge production and acquisition through what one sees suggests a physical vision as opposed to a mental vision. Mental vision has transformative possibilities that should be promoted in oral cultures such as those found in many African societies.

In societies in which cultural production is realized primarily through orature, the ability to engage in the production of individual and collective mental imagery in learning is superior to visual/physical abilities. This process of cultural communication is eschewed in many health programs being implemented today in most African countries. Instead of focusing on encouraging the production of mental vision that engages individuals by affirming their own space and voice, institutions of higher learning (which for the most part provide training instead of education), as well as development agencies, have naturalized and reified the production of standardized learning based on physical vision. The result is a push for physical learning, such as the use of transparencies and slide projectors as the ultimate form of sharing and communicating knowledge based culturally on philosophy and practice. In fact, some institutions in both Northern and Southern nations have gone so far as to require that those who share knowledge, whether students making classroom presentations or professionals presenting conference papers, use physical/visual materials as the primary tool of communication, with the speaker's voice serving only a secondary function.

This form of learning has been promoted even though very few educators can effectively and efficiently use slides, transparencies, and other materials to engage their audiences in the production and acquisition of knowledge. For the majority, such presentations have become a form of standardized mediocrity; the speaker no longer has to aspire toward acquiring a voice that can transport the audience and/or student to undertake an independent cultural journey that leads to production of meaning. Rather, professionals have settled for a uniform, often Western- and male-centered meaning—the ultimate form of what Freire (1973) refers to as "castration of curiosity" in learners. The paradox in this case becomes evident in how we reward speakers and affirm leadership in education. In certain circumstances, it is the individual who is able to "stand and deliver," in the absence of visual support, who is worthy of recognition. Evidence of this tradition abounds among people of African descent.

> The scholar, rhetorician, or historian who undertakes an analysis of the Black past without recognizing the significance of vocal expression as a transforming agent is treading on intellectual quicksand. . . . What is clear is that leaders who articulated and articulate the grievances felt by the masses have always understood the power of the word in the Black

community. . . . Their emergence has always been predicated upon the power of the spoken word. (Asante, 1987, p. 86)

The power of the spoken word has always been recognized by Africans as the hallmark of the varied interpretations and value of storytelling. Such interpretations are sometimes encoded in songs of a story, such that the wisdom of the story is recalled in the song. The Edos of Nigeria always begin a story by singing a song that captures the spirit and the message of the story. Songs and dances are central to nearly all Edo rituals celebrating rain, birth, circumcision, and marriage, as well as funerals and more ordinary ceremonies. Songs and dances are not just decorative additions to an occasion; they are an integral part of the conversation, the drinking session, the ritual, the ceremony (Thiong'O, 1986).

Although songs and dances are central to the Edo form of cultural production, individuals need certain skills to navigate the terrain of meanings and codes enshrined in the cultural landscape. Such skills are often acquired through experiential education and training. Indifferent and sometimes oblivious to the significance of songs and dances, as well as storytelling, in many African countries, Westernized/Eurocentric intellectuals have often engaged themselves in these media of expression even though they have no training, skills, or understanding of these forms of cultural production. Such culture-effacing acts are an extension of the belief that orature/oracy as a form of cultural production is simplistic, premodern, and easily engaged in by anyone with training in the more "complex" (written tradition) form of cultural production. Untrained in oral communication, and acting from their incorrect perceptions of the simplicity of the oral genre, these individuals produce simple stories and songs that defy cultural codes, interpretations, and meanings. Chinweizu, Jemie, and Madubuike (1983), in their classic book *Toward the Decolonization of African Literature,* challenge the prejudices that are often espoused by Eurocentrists when evaluating African literature and oral tradition:

In evaluating African literature and matters related to it, they [Eurocentrists] start out by taking outstanding written material from Europe as their standards; they gather whatever African material

> they find convenient, usually of middling quality or worse, and compare them adversely with the best from Europe, and thereby unctuously confirm themselves in their initial prejudice that Europe is "good" and Africa is "bad." When it comes to the African oral tradition, their anti-African prejudice is reinforced by their anti-oral prejudice. They therefore gather the most grossly inadequate versions of African oral material they can find, and proceed, once again, to unctuously confirm themselves in their double-barrelled prejudice against things both African and oral. (p. 87)

The use of language in any culture is designed to mirror the worldview of the culture. It is often suggested that African languages have limitations in their usage, but this is a myopic conclusion that uses Western standards to evaluate the lexical functions of all languages and their cultural relevancies. According to Chinweizu et al. (1983), the "issue of parity and reciprocity has implications for the matter of making comparisons between the oral and written modes. Cognizance ought to be taken of the diversity of genres within the oral and the written forms, so that only comparable forms are compared" (p. 35). The possibilities of the oral genre include the mystification of reality and the reality of myths, the spontaneity of communication and communicating spontaneously, and the extension of the interpretive potentials of cultural codes and meanings even when invoked for the first time.

A common theme in the stories of African cultures is the interaction between animate and inanimate objects. This has been demonstrated in the fictional works of Wole Soyinka and Ben Okri, among others, in which people assume animal functions and roles and vice versa. Trees and other inanimate objects can communicate verbally. Earthly phenomena such as animal forms and their peculiarities are explained in fables.

Knowledge is culturally produced through forms of direct and indirect exchange between parents and children, teachers and students, and speakers and audiences. For example, the colonial mentality of expecting non-Western cultures to embrace Western paradigms without critically analyzing them creates a lose/lose situation. To suggest that non-Western cultures should play a catch-up game with the West is to suggest that their cultural values and production could never equate with "progress." Meanwhile, the West continues to devise new markers for "progress," from *savage* to *underdevelopment/development*, and now *globalization.*

This relationship of the West to the rest of us can be illustrated by the relationship between the egg and the coconut—it does not matter whether the egg falls on the coconut or the coconut falls on the egg, it is the egg that will break. The coconut and egg represent different identities that, allowing for some possibilities of hybridization, in principle affirm each other's particular space. Considered side by side, they represent different forms of cultural production and meaning on the global landscape. They echo the philosophy that searches for multiple truths because when one thing stands, another thing stands beside it. Neither the egg nor the coconut is static in its cultural representation. In other words, whereas a culture may symbolize the egg in one instance, in another it may be the coconut. For example, although many African cultural codes and meanings (the coconut) were impervious to assault during colonialism and postcolonialism (i.e., the introduction of traditional medicine), these same societies have yielded (the egg) to the adoption and often valorization of non-African languages for political, educational, personal, and business/market exchanges. By the same token, although the Western cultures have maintained their religious traditions (the coconut), these same cultures have yielded (the egg) some formal codes and are now being influenced by music and clothing constructed by ethnic minorities.

The victor in the cultural clash of such forms of knowledge acquisition becomes a part of a culture and establishes the initial basis upon which subsequent opinions are formulated, attitudes and values developed, inquisitions made, and knowledge produced. The use of adages and proverbs is usually the hallmark of changes in education and cultural codes in traditional settings. It is very important for the rest of us to understand the full ramification of undue reliance on Western paradigms for the meaning of progress. There are long-term, irreversible consequences for continuing to operate under Western hegemonic influences, because "no one said a child should not have big teeth as long as he or she has lips big enough to cover them." For example, in 1973 Robert McNamara, president of the World Bank, declared that GNP as a singular measure of development has exacerbated inequalities in income distribution, because more and more people become poorer as GNP grows (Illich, 1992). In other words, development as conceived in the West has led to regression in the standard of living in Southern nations.

Two decades after the realization of the failure of development concept, and four years after the U.N. Development Programme's (1993) *Human Development Report* called for the inclusion and emphasis of noneconomic indicators (e.g., food security and status of women) in measuring progress, the implementation of the development concept as informed by the dominant paradigm continues to flourish in Southern nations. Although World Bank and U.N. Development Programme reports have questioned the validity of equating development/GNP with progress, they have still failed to centralize cultural production and meaning at the core of the measurement of progress.

If the importance of a cultural domain affects the lexical complexity of that domain, then the absence of words to delineate family kinship along biological lines in many African cultures is of lexical significance. According to W. Kamau (personal communication, 1993), among the Kikuyus of Kenya, the first male child (I do not say "first son" because the terms *son* and *daughter* resonate with parent-child closure that does not allow for the inclusion of other members of the extended family in the rearing of the child) bears the name of his paternal grandfather and the first female child bears the name of the paternal grandmother. The second male child bears the name of the maternal grandfather, and the second female child bears the name of the maternal grandmother. The relationships that exist between children and grandparents in this context are rooted in a strong belief that the future (our children) is an extension of the past (our parents). A grandparent becomes closely bonded with his or her rebirth (the grandchild) and assumes unflinching and unwavering personal responsibility toward the child. The child is often referred to in the name and designation of his or her grandparent, whose life the child is on earth to relive. The child soon begins to internalize the role, persona, and values of the grandparent in a psychologically preordained role-modeling relationship. In most cases, according to Kamau, the child begins to manifest certain physical and behavioral traits of the grandparent—a powerful form of family and cultural production and reproduction.

Among the Kikuyus, these cultural codes and meanings are critical for couples' decisions regarding the number of children they desire (a goal for family planning programs) and the number of children they have in the process of seeking to balance the gender representations of the children as a fulfillment of their cultural expressions. Such cultural fulfillment may result in undue pressure on a couple, especially the wife, to have at least two boys and two girls. However, the bonding, psychogenealogical extension, and family and cultural reproductions are values and nurturing that symbiotically benefit the children and parents in their collective growth and transformation. These collective experiences, which are not always quantifiable—nor should they be—are the hallmark of the sustenance of the extended family in Africa.

The fact that many relatives are referred to as brothers and sisters (even though these include those who would be considered nephews, nieces, and cousins in Western cultures) is often believed to be an example of the limitation of languages in African cultures. The possibility that this way of speaking is deliberately constructed to capture the closeness and bonding that typifies the sibling relationship is rarely entertained. To learn that there is a difference between one's brothers/sisters and one's cousins and other so-called distant relations is to learn about developing cognitive and affective distance in the way one relates to those relatives. Among the Edos of Nigeria, where children are familiar only with the concept of brothers and sisters, there is a type of closeness and reciprocal responsibility peculiar to the culture that is theirs to value. In fact, the concept of brothers and sisters in the African context is one of the most important factors in the maintenance and sustenance of extended family in Africa.

Moreover, the term *extended family* suggests that the Westernized nuclear family is the norm. When the extended family is used as the norm, situating it at the center instead of the margin, the Western family becomes the alternative type of family, the "constricted family." When I was growing up in Nigeria, I always knew that my nephew was my brother. Upon coming to the United States for "training," I began to refer to my brother by the Western designation (my nephew). As time progressed, I began to experience some level of inexplicable mental distance that was never the case in Nigeria. It was as though I suddenly discovered that my brother was adopted by my parents, but unfortunately my parents were not with me to buffer the shock and confusion that followed this discovery. It was up to me alone to overcome the irrelevance of the Western genealogical demarcation, as it were, and hold on to the wisdom of my parents and my culture. I had to make a conscious effort to revert to referring to my brother as my brother.

I would argue that our foremothers and forefathers intentionally left out words and delineators that could potentially distance relatives. Such affirmative vision speaks to the cultural sophistication and pragmatism of Africans in the production of knowledge, with its carefully constructed cultural codes and meanings. Of course, for Eurocentrists, to affirm this is to subscribe to an episteme that is not consistent with or may be superior to that of the West. One does not have to understand or logically follow cultural codes or expressions to affirm and respect their legitimating values. After all, everyday language usage that defies logic has always influenced the interpretive meanings and visual imagery given to life experience. For example, we speak of *sunrise* and *sunset,* although these terms tend to suggest that the world is flat rather than that the earth spins in its orbit around the sun. This has never stopped people from using these expressions or led them to change their value and meaning, even though perhaps more accurate terms would be *earthrise* and *earthset.*

Cultural practices relating to patterns of knowledge production and acquisition, in this case oral tradition, must be seriously considered in health communication interventions in cultures in which orature is the primary basis of communication. Health communication projects conducted in Africa to date have tended to operate on three key assumptions:

1. Health information can reach the populace through the media.
2. This health information can change negative health practices if the population has the requisite health knowledge. Therefore, the health information should focus on the acquisition of the relevant health knowledge.
3. If the people do not acquire the relevant health information, it means that their skills for acquiring these messages must be developed. This often translates to development of literacy programs for the target population. In fact, literacy is being hailed as the key to improving the health conditions of Africans.

The problem with these operational assumptions is that they place all of the responsibility for program outcomes on the actions or inaction of the people in the target communities. Therefore, if a program fails, it is always reasoned that the target community lacked the requisite knowledge and/or motivation to initiate the expected health actions that would lead to positive health outcomes. The health interventionists are absolved of any responsibility and accountability for the failure of the program participants to attain the expected health outcomes. Eurocentrists refuse to interrogate their complicity in the formation and imposition of their cultural hegemony on Others as constructed in the interplay of language and difference (Giroux, 1992). One of the manifestations of this interplay is the proliferation of adult literacy programs in Africa.

## Literacy and Educational Interventions

Unfortunately, literacy has been equated with education and, ultimately, stages and levels of development. Although literacy is usually a by-product of Western formal education, education (acquisition of the skills and information needed to make informed decisions) is not always the outcome of literacy. In fact, some of the traditional literacy programs were designed to provide unsuspecting consumers with the skills to understand and purchase certain advertised products. This is not surprising, given that literacy is believed to be the springboard to national development.

The misguided notion of literacy as a precursor for national development is based on Anderson's (1966) claim that a society requires a 40% adult literacy rate for economic "takeoff" (cited in Street, 1984). This paradigm has resulted in the widespread development and promotion of adult literacy programs, particularly in Southern nations. This practice continues today, in light of the fact that people tend to lose literacy skills if their daily engagements do not involve reading and/or writing. In fact, a number of the illiterate adults in some African countries today were once able to read and write as a result of completing primary school education. The ability to read and write is like many other skills in that you can learn it, but if you do not use it, you lose it. Thus most of the current literacy programs are simply reinventing the wheel—or, worse yet, they are reinventing the flat tire.

UNESCO attempted to improve the sustainability of literacy skills by creating what it called a "literacy environment" (Street, 1984). This simply meant that the environment of a community would be transformed to fit the needs and desires of those promoting the literacy program, rather than the program's being modified to fit with the community environment. Challenging UNESCO and others who perpetrate this neocolonial violence on Southern nations, Freire (1973) and some other cultural workers have proposed adult literacy programs that engage the participants as subjects rather than objects. Using this approach, participants are engaged in the construction of sociopolitical issues that shape their collective reality, in a "process of consciencization." In Freire's adult literacy model, the participants are exposed to social and political issues that affect them so that they can become involved and have input into the decisions that affect them. "No program of literacy-training can exist—as the naive claim—which is not connected with the work of human beings, their technical proficiency, their view of the world" (Freire, 1973, p. 157), because "literacy involves not just the reading of the word, but also the reading of the World" (Freire, 1993, p. 59).

Even when the goal of a literacy program is sensitive to the cultural reality of the people the program is designed to benefit, the methods and techniques of implementation are often not culturally sensitive. In this respect, it is important to examine the methods employed in health communications. Specifically, we should examine the level of congruence between the traditional mode of learning (oral—mouth to ear) and the Western mode of learning (visual—eye to object). In other words, to what degree does the use of posters and flyers, which are visually dependent, conflict with the traditional method of learning in an oral tradition? Literacy is critical to the degree that it problematizes the very structure and practice of representation by focusing attention on the fact that meaning is not fixed and that to be literate is to undertake a dialogue with others who speak from different histories, locations, and experiences (Giroux, 1992). Literacy is yet another development index that has been used to pursue the notion of universal truths.

A major problem in the planning and development of health programs has been the preoccupation with seeking a universal solution.

This fixation has resulted in the misrepresentation of the diverse cultural realities of Africans, as though they are monolithic. As Freire (1970) notes:

> One of the characteristics of oppressive cultural action which is almost never perceived by the dedicated but naive professionals who are involved is the emphasis on a focalized view of problems rather than on seeing them as dimensions of a totality. In "community development" projects the more a region or area is broken down into "local communities," without the study of these communities both as totalities in themselves and as part of another totality (the area, region, and so forth)—which in its turn is a part of a still larger totality (the nation, as part of the continental totality)—the more alienation is intensified. (p. 138)

On the issue of universal truth espoused in the dominant paradigm, Faundez comments, "Whereas Europeans try to discover what there is in *common*, and that becomes the essential for them, for me the essential is the 'differences,' and, since each time I discover differences, each time I become more aware of how little I know" (in Freire & Faundez, 1989, p. 32).

As a consultant to the World Health Organization in 1991, I was asked to develop a health education curriculum in Geneva (this request did not come from the Division of Health Education). This guideline was to be used in the development of health curricula in several African countries, without the involvement of participants from those countries. I protested and registered my objection to being a party to a process that totally disempowers the teachers, administrators, and students in these countries. Such is a Geneva hegemony (in spite of the fact that some WHO programs tend to be progressive) that marginalizes Africans by denying them the opportunity to be subjects and actors in the systematization of educational processes that will shape their future. This sophisticated form of colonization is practiced by using a credentialed member of the marginalized group to sustain Western hegemony in the name of inclusion and pluralism. It has become a common practice for national and international institutions to recruit unsuspecting credentialed Others (including Third World nationals and members of minority groups in the First World) to pursue and promote what are believed to be universal solutions to the problems of the Others' people. Although an increase in the representation and involvement of disenfranchised Others is welcome, it does not absolve decision makers of their responsibility to examine their complicitous actions/inactions and myopic approaches. Neither should these practices continue to exclude the participation of Others in the production of knowledge and cultural identity.

## Conclusion

Cultural sensitivity in health promotion, education, and development programs can be realized only when we centralize the cultural experiences of those who have hitherto been marginalized in the production of knowledge and cultural identity. To be specific, it is counterproductive to target individuals for most health risk reduction efforts without considering the effects of those individuals' cultures, languages, and environments. Educators must use source expertise to manipulate the social, political, and environmental forces that influence health behavior within the context of particular cultures (Airhihenbuwa, DiClemente, Wingood, & Lowe, 1992). However, the onus of manipulating these environmental forces must not rest solely on the people targeted for health promotion and disease prevention. Ultimately, the source experts are catalysts; they must be seen as symbolic of the resolve and potential of the groups they represent, not as exceptions. The true experts in the methods of the production and acquisition of knowledge in a culture are the people themselves. In Chapter 3, I present a cultural model and examples of its application to various population groups.

# 3

# Developing Culturally Appropriate Health Programs

> How we view ourselves, our environment even, is very much dependent on where we stand in relationship to imperialism in its colonial and neo-colonial stages; that if we are to do anything about our individual and collective being today, then we have to coldly and consciously look at what imperialism has been doing to us and to our view of ourselves in the universe.
>
> *Ngugi Wa Thiong'O, Decolonizing the Mind, 1986*

The focus on primary health care as the international road map to universal health coverage commonly referred to as the Alma-Ata Declaration, and subsequently the African ministers of health's introduction of a cost-effective framework for financing primary health care known as the Bamako Initiative, placed the emphasis in global health improvement on primary health care. Public health observers with commitment to improving health in Southern nations have embraced this focus as realistic and appropriate. There is no single strategy for understanding complex health problems, but an understanding of

AUTHOR'S NOTE: This chapter is an expanded version of my article "Health Promotion for Child Survival in Africa: Implications for Cultural Appropriateness," *International Journal of Health Education, 12*(3), 10-15. Copyright © 1993 by the International Union for Health Promotion and Education. Used by permission.

the complexity of the problems is a prerequisite of the proposal of effective solutions. It is more effective to adapt preventive health programs to fit community needs and cultural contexts than the reverse, hence the need to ensure that health promotion programs are culturally appropriate. Although several health education/promotion models/frameworks are currently being used in the planning, implementation, and evaluation of preventive health programs, none seems to centralize culture as a critical force in the prevention of disease and the promotion of health.

The training of any person for an occupation requires an understanding of culture as a superstructure that can maintain "remnants" of the past alive in the substructure undergoing revolutionary transformation and of the occupation itself as an instrument for the transformation of culture (Freire, 1973). Health beliefs and actions should be examined within the context of culture, history, and politics. In this chapter I present the PEN-3 model, a conceptual model used in the planning and development of culturally appropriate health education/promotion programs (Airhihenbuwa, 1989b, 1990-1991, 1992). To illustrate the model, I discuss its application to child survival interventions in Nigeria. The version of the model presented here is a slight modification of the original.

## Background on Health Education Approaches

Among approaches to health education/promotion and disease prevention, the self-empowerment method is believed to be more encompassing and more effective than preventive-medical or radical-political approaches. The preventive-medical approach focuses on influencing individual decisions leading to the adoption of positive health behaviors, whereas the radical-political approach focuses on manipulating the social and political environment so as to tackle ill health at its foundation (Tones, Tilford, & Robinson, 1991, pp. 1-16). The preventive-medical approach has a tendency to blame the victim; the radical-political approach can be biased toward the interests and priorities of the health interventionists, even when such interests and priorities are at variance with those of the target community. The self-empowerment approach facilitates choices for individuals and communities within the context of the sociocultural and political environment. This is accomplished through the supplementation of health knowledge acquisition with values clarification and practice skills in decision making through nontraditional teaching methods. Thus the self-empowerment method draws on the positive elements of both the preventive-medical and the radical-political approaches (Tones et al., 1991). However, a striking but limiting feature of the self-empowerment approach is the emphasis on *self.* Such emphasis places the onus of responsibility for health behavior outcome on the individual—a limitation shared with the preventive-medical approach. Given this limitation, I use the term *cultural empowerment* here to extend the possibilities of the empowerment approach. Cultural empowerment takes into account how health knowledge, beliefs, and actions are produced and interpreted at both micro (individual, family, and community/grassroots) and macro (national and international power and politics) levels. Thus the decision making of individuals and families must be situated within its proper political, historical, and cultural context.

*Cultural sensitivity,* in health promotion and behavior change programs, refers to the development and adaptation of programs so that they are situated within appropriate cultural frameworks rather than the Western so-called scientific culture within which most health and development programs are planned, implemented, and evaluated. Health results from a process of adaptation. It is the result not of instinct but of an autonomous yet culturally shaped reaction to socially created reality (Illich, 1976).

When present values and practices are not seriously considered in health and development programs, their usefulness within the cultural context of African communities is at best questionable. Thus to locate culture at the core of health education/promotion programs is to require a thorough examination and understanding of the historicity within the cultural and political context of present health beliefs and actions of a people. This is a process of cultural empowerment.

This process of empowering individuals in health education programming is often based on the assumption that individuals, primarily because of their limited economic resources, are powerless. Eurocentrists often consider silence, which makes most Westerners uncomfortable, to indicate voicelessness and weakness. They thus believe that knowledge can be measured using economic/development indices such as income level and fluency in a Western language. Failing to recognize that knowledge born of the Western economic/developmental praxis carries questionable values and biases that marginalize traditional and local knowledge, Eurocentrists introduced the notion of empowerment in a form of "participation" to legitimate the development concept (Rahnema, 1992). The authoritarian connotation of participation obviously reduces it to a presence of the popular classes in the administration of development programs (Freire, 1993). This silencing of Others through development participation foregrounds the impetus for the construction of a culturally appropriate programmatic framework for health promotion programs in Africa. This process, known as PEN-3, has been employed to guide workshops on child survival in Nigeria as well as workshops on AIDS and diet and exercise among African Americans.

## The PEN-3 Model

Any conceptual approach for health promotion programs should be anchored in a dialogic process that allows members of the targeted culture to address cultural sensitivity and cultural appropriateness in program development. Although I refer to PEN-3 as a model, my intent is not for it to be applied in some prefabricated box or matrix but for it to offer a space within which cultural codes and meanings can be centralized in the development, implementation, and evaluation of health promotion programs.

The PEN-3 model allows the kind of flexibility that encourages intracultural diversity such that the process should be engaged each time a program is conceived. Health workers should employ a dialogic process that ensures affirmation of different cultural expressions in specific locations. Moreover, this method also challenges health and cultural workers to address health issues at the macro (policy, government, societal, and international) level as well as the traditional micro level of health program interventions. The utility of this method therefore relates to its amenability to modification and extension of its limits and possibilities such that the production and acquisition of knowledge in the target culture is sensitively and sensibly represented in the project. In addition, this method incorporates existing models/theories and frameworks in health education while drawing on theory and application in cultural studies. Thus PEN-3 consists of three dimensions of health beliefs and behavior that are dynamically interrelated and interdependent: health education, educational diagnosis of health behavior, and cultural appropriateness of health behavior.

The PEN-3 model is illustrated in Figure 3.1, which lists the three categories (according to the acronym PEN) within each of the three dimensions. The first dimension of the PEN-3 model is health education, the three categories of which are person, extended family, and neighborhood.

*Person.* Health education is committed to the health of all. To this end, individuals should be empowered to make informed health decisions appropriate to their roles in their families and communities.

*Extended family.* Health education is concerned not only with the immediate, nuclear family but also with extended kin. Such a focus on the extended family should also take into account family lineage (e.g., patrilinear or matrilinear). However, when a program is designed to target a particular member of the family (e.g., the mother), the individual should become the focus of the study and must be so recognized. Such recognition must be noted within the context of the individual's environment.

*Neighborhood.* Health education is committed to promoting health and preventing disease in neighborhoods and communities. Involvement of community members and their leaders becomes critical in the provision of culturally appropriate health programs. In fact, because community leadership often defines community boundaries, it is critical for leaders to define what constitutes their community or neighborhood at the beginning of a project.

The second dimension of PEN-3 is the educational diagnosis of health behavior. Educational diagnosis has been used by researchers to attempt determination of the factors that influence individual, family, and/or community health actions. The three predominant

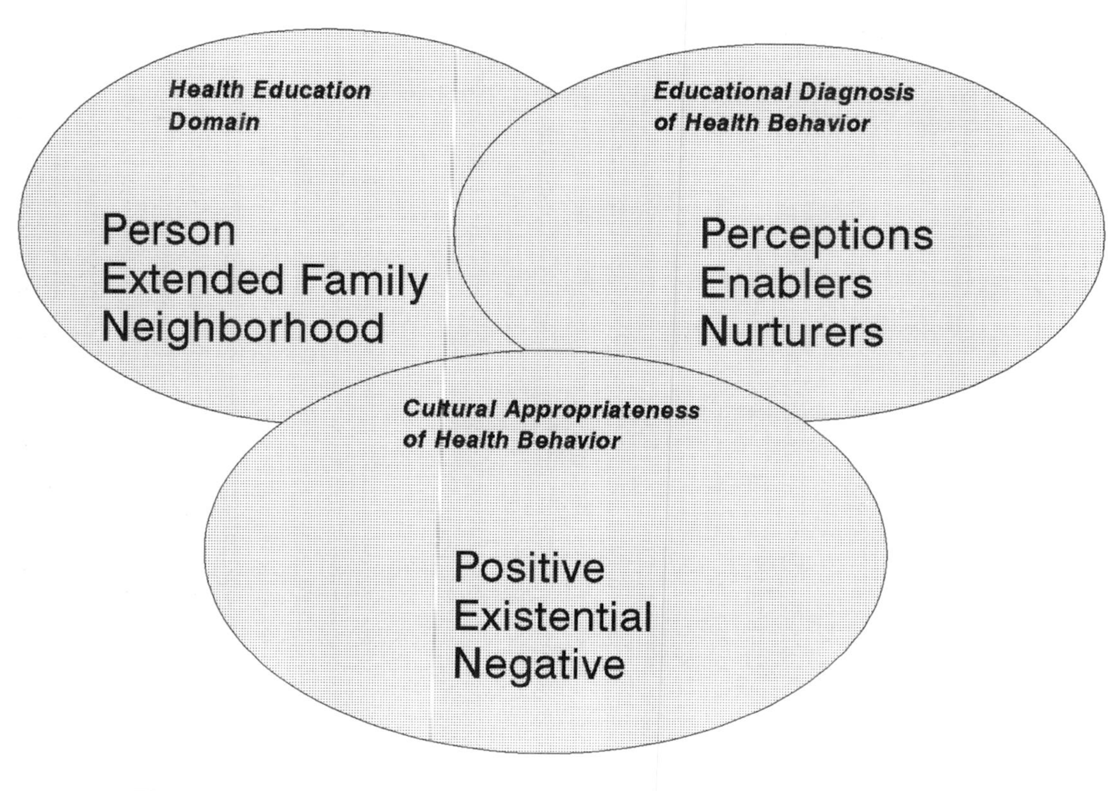


**Figure 3.1.** The PEN-3 Model

models or frameworks that have been used in understanding and predicting health-related behaviors are the health belief model (Rosenstock, 1974), Fishbein and Ajzen's (1975) theory of reasoned action, and the PRECEDE framework (Mullen, Hersey, & Iverson, 1987). Influenced by Kurt Lewin's (1947) "life space" notion, the health belief model deals with individuals' perceptions of their susceptibility to disease and of the severity of their diseases as predictors of their health actions. Fishbein and Ajzen's theory of reasoned action postulates that behavioral intention is a function of attitude toward performance of an impending behavior reinforced by feedback from significant others. The PRECEDE-PROCEED framework (Green & Kreuter, 1991) deals with how to identify, change/modify, and evaluate which health-related and non-health-related behaviors are most important and changeable, taking into account personal, family, community, and environmental factors.

This dimension of PEN-3 has evolved from the confluence of the three aforementioned models of health education. However, it is important to note that culture has no central role in educational diagnosis in these earlier models. PEN-3 therefore extends the possibilities of this dimension as advanced in previous health education models and frameworks by placing culture at the core of health promotion and disease prevention programs. The factors in the second dimension of the PEN-3 approach are perceptions, enablers, and nurturers.

*Perceptions.* Perceptions comprise the knowledge, attitudes, values, and beliefs, within a cultural context, that may facilitate or hinder personal, family, and community motivation to change. For example, some Nigerian mothers believe that a healthy child does not need to be protected against illness, and this may affect immunization programs, because preventive injections have always been considered treatment. Or, for instance, if there is a cultural belief that consuming sweet foods causes diarrhea (a belief held by the Edos, Yorubas, and Igbos of Nigeria), it will be a serious challenge to promote the use of homemade oral rehydration solutions, which contain sugar, as therapy for diarrhea. Existing perceptions can lead to the need to resolve conflicts that might arise in people's minds, because to them it might seem as though the causative agent of a disease is also its cure. For example, when African Americans have answered yes to the question "Can someone get AIDS from donating blood?" some researchers have misinterpreted this to mean they have poor AIDS knowledge. In fact, this response sometimes indicates a strong negative distrust of White health care providers, reflecting a belief that they may intentionally infect Blacks with the AIDS virus—a perception that is a legacy of the Tuskegee syphilis experiments and ongoing racism in general. In regard to differences in perception of body weight between African Americans and Whites, several researchers have reported that being overweight is not necessarily associated with negative body image for many African Americans (e.g., Desmond, Price, Hallinan, & Smith, 1989; Kumanyika, Wilson, & Guilford-Davenport, 1993). African Americans who are heavy or of normal weight are likely to perceive themselves as thinner than are their White counterparts. In fact, in one study, 40% of African American women who were classified as overweight considered their figures attractive or very attractive. However, such perceptions about body image should not compromise the seriousness of obesity as a predisposing factor to chronic degenerative conditions such as type II diabetes and heart disease.

*Enablers.* Enablers are cultural, societal, systematic, or structural influences or forces that may enhance or be barriers to change, such as the availability of resources, accessibility, referrals, employers, government officials, skills, and types of services (e.g., traditional medicine). At a child survival workshop in Nigeria, several mothers cited being asked to pay for the treatment of abscesses (a side effect of vaccination) as a major reason for not taking their children for immunization through the Expanded Program on Immunization (EPI), even though they know the injections are free. Paulo Freire discovered that mothers' reluctance and/or refusal to give eggs to their children started when colonial settlers told the indigenes that eggs were bad for them (the indigenes), so that eggs would be sold cheaply (because they were of little use to those who produced them) to the colonizers (in Freire & Faundez, 1989). Finally, opportunity costs are always an important factor to be considered in the planning and implementation of health intervention programs for African American communities.

*Nurturers.* Another important element is the degree to which health beliefs, attitudes, and actions are influenced and mediated, or nurtured, by extended family, kin, friends, peers, and the community. For example, the fact that older siblings who were never immunized are in good health tends to suggest to some grandparents that EPI and other modern preventive actions against childhood diseases are unwarranted for their younger grandchildren. The concept of nurturers emphasizes the importance of increasing significantly the number of African Americans in the health professions who understand and respect African American culture and communities. It is also important to promote an understanding of cultural beliefs and practices among non-African Americans. For example, because of the disproportionately high level of cardiovascular disease in the African American population, special emphasis has been placed on eating practices and weight control. Because food is a cultural symbol and eating is a symbolic act through which people communicate, perpetuate, and develop their knowledge and attitudes toward life, an understanding of cultural influences on eating habits is essential for the health educator who wants to provide realistic educational interventions designed to modify dietary practices (Kaufman-Kurzrock, 1989).

The third and most critical dimension of the PEN-3 model is the cultural appropriateness of health behavior. This dimension is pivotal to the development of a culturally sensitive health education program. This dimension situates culture in dynamic and interacting forces that manifest themselves in individual, family, and community behavior. Each of these three dimensions can relate to perceptions, enablers, and nurturers within their historical and cultural contexts. This final dimension consists of the categories of positive, existential, and negative behaviors.

*Positive behaviors.* These are behaviors that are based on health beliefs and actions that are known to be beneficial and must be encouraged. These behaviors are critical in the empowerment of persons, extended families, and neighborhoods. Affirmation of these behaviors is critical to program success and sustainability, particularly because they are examples of these cultures' contributions to the global production of knowledge and meaning. Examples include the promotion of such traditional practices as breast-feeding and the eating of green vegetables. There is a tendency on the part of upwardly mobile African American professionals to disengage slowly from eating green vegetables, as was done traditionally, because such foods are not believed to be associated with progress and affluence.

*Existential behaviors.* Existential behaviors comprise those cultural beliefs, practices, and/or behaviors that are indigenous to a group and have no harmful health consequences, and thus need not be targeted for change and should not be blamed for program failure simply because they are ill understood. An example is the use of palm oil and indigo as a soothing lotion for a child with measles. Another example is the placing of an amulet around a child's neck to ward off evil spirits. In fact, some physicians have actually used this practice with their pediatric patients, telling them that only the physicians may remove the amulets. This helps to guarantee that patients will return for follow-up visits.

Public health educators should address what *is* and not what *ought to be.* They should refrain from moralizing over behaviors that are unfamiliar to them and that they do not understand. The programmatic thrust of public health should be to address what is in terms of matching intervention with current health practices, such as sexual activities among teenagers, rather than what ought to be, such as abstinence. Understanding these existential beliefs is where African American theoreticians have made significant contributions. For example, these researchers link African American lifestyles, at least in part, with African values to produce a holistic worldview, as opposed to an abstract construction of personality assessment that sees the individual as pathologic.

*Negative behaviors.* Negative behaviors are based on health beliefs and actions that are known to be harmful to health: Health providers must therefore examine and understand them within their cultural, historical, and political contexts before attempting to change them. Examples of negative behaviors include the withholding of fluid from a victim of diarrhea and unprotected sexual intercourse.

In PEN-3, the *Es*—extended family, enablers, and existential behaviors—are the most powerful influences on and for cultural production. The enablers speak to power, politics, and history; the existential speaks to affirmation of humanity and cultural empowerment; and extended family speaks to the vitality of sustained positive traditions and influence as well as a major contribution to global production of knowledge, meaning, and interpretation. The dynamic interrelatedness of these three levels must be balanced to demonstrate the degree to which politics, policy, power, and culture shape and are being shaped by individuals and the family.

Health education programs involve health beliefs and behaviors. These programs must reflect the cultural perspectives of the people for whom they are designed. Health educators should focus on both positive (cultural empowerment process) and negative behaviors in a health program. Very often, too much attention is focused on negative behaviors, with few or no rewards offered for positive behaviors. In some instances, educators arrogantly blame the failure to change negative behaviors on the presence of existential behaviors.

The process of culturalizing health knowledge, attitudes, and practices does not assume that people are powerless or ignorant. The process affirms diversity in the way people construct their individual and collective realities within the possibilities of their locations. What is positive or negative cannot be based on a universal notion promoted in economic development. In fact, the process challenges the shortcomings of empowerment as advanced in the economic/development paradigm. Rahnema (1992) illustrates these shortcomings in the following:

> When A considers it essential for B to be empowered, A assumes not only that B has no power—or does not have the right kind of power—but also that A has the secret formula of a power to which B has to be initiated. In the current *participatory ideology,* this formula is, in fact, nothing but a revised version of state power, or what could be called fear-power. The crux of the matter is that populations actually subjected to this fear-power are not at all powerless. (p. 123; emphasis added)

## Implementation of Child Survival Programs

The PEN-3 model was operationalized at the African Regional Child Survival Workshop in Nigeria, June-July 1990, and subsequently at the training of trainers workshop for Africare and the Imo (Nigeria)

State Ministry of Health. A total of 20 participants from 10 different African countries representing 10 private voluntary organizations with child survival projects were assigned to four intervention groups—oral rehydration therapy (ORT), EPI, nutrition, and high-risk birth. On the basis of their child survival field experiences, each group developed a list of reported positive, existential, and negative health beliefs related to their assigned interventions. These health beliefs reflected the perceptions, enablers, and nurturers of members of the communities for whom the child survival projects were designed. With the information generated on positive, existential, and negative health beliefs, each intervention group developed a list of interview questions (according to perceptions, enablers, and nurturers) for one of four preselected segments of the community. The four segments of the community that were interviewed were mothers, village health workers, traditional leaders, and local government representatives. Information about child survival interventions was obtained from the community on perceptions (beliefs related to knowledge, attitudes, and practices), enablers (culture, structure, skills, and resources necessary for health actions), and nurturers (family, kin, and friend reinforcement for health beliefs and practices). The participants then classified the items into positive, existential, and negative health beliefs and practices so as to delineate appropriately the focus for health promotion and disease prevention in the community.

At the end of the first workshop, a second was held with the staff of the Ministry of Health who provide training for the village health workers in the area. At this second workshop, the information generated at the first was used to classify health beliefs into two categories. Listed below are the beliefs that were identified under the dimension of cultural appropriateness of health behavior. Each belief/practice is labeled either T, for a long-term health belief that is deeply rooted in the tradition and culture, or R, for a recent and short-term health belief that may or may not become part of long-term tradition.

**Positive: Cultural Empowerment**

1. The idea of taking fluids during illness is acceptable. T

2. The community noticed a decline in diarrhea morbidity/mortality with ORT usage. R
3. Community leaders are willing and able to take the lead as change agents. T
4. The giving of plantain porridge to children who have diarrhea is acceptable. T
5. The giving of pap and/or coconut juice to children who have diarrhea is acceptable. T
6. Sexual abstinence during pregnancy reduces the incidence of pelvic inflammatory disease. T

## Existential: No Threat to Health

1. Beads around a child's wrist and/or ankle will ward off evil spirits. T
2. Postpartum sexual abstinence prevents semen from mixing with breast milk. T
3. Palm oil and indigo serve as a good soothing lotion for measles. T
4. Families should have a lot of children because of high child mortality rates. R
5. Women should have all the children that God gives them. T

## Negative: Threat to Health

1. Male dominance inhibits necessary female participation. T/R
2. Feeding a child certain foods, such as eggs and meat, causes the child to steal. T
3. Eating sugar and other sweet foods causes diarrhea. T
4. Medicine is needed for diarrhea, and ORT is not medicine. R
5. Babies with diarrhea must not be breast-fed. T
6. A healthy child does not need health care; therefore, immunization is unnecessary. T
7. Immunization may cause disability and/or death in a child. R
8. Because older, living, healthy siblings were not immunized, there is no reason to immunize infants. R
9. Contraceptives and tetanus toxoid cause sterility. R
10. A pregnant woman's eating eggs, meat, or chicken causes her baby to be too big to deliver normally. T
11. Taking fluids during diarrhea will prolong diarrhea and/or will result in the development of worms. T

The health workers then conducted a workshop with the village health workers to discuss these health beliefs, particularly those that are rooted in tradition and culture. It should be noted that the above dichotomy does not represent a static classification. This classification was provided by health workers who train the village health workers. What is traditional or recent may vary from one location to another.

## Application of the Model

In the development of programs that fit in with a community's existing beliefs and practices, the PEN-3 model can be utilized as illustrated by the steps taken in the workshops described above. In the first phase, the program planners must determine whether the emphasis of the program will be on the person, the extended family, or the neighborhood (health education), realizing that these are not mutually exclusive categories. In the second phase, the planners should explore (through surveys and/or interviews) the beliefs and practices related to perceptions, enablers, and nurturers (educational diagnosis of health behavior). Such examinations will relate to a particular health problem in different segments of the family or community. On the basis of the information generated, in the third phase the planners should categorize the different beliefs and practices found into positive, existential, and negative beliefs (cultural appropriateness of health behavior). Finally, with the assistance and guidance of community health workers, the planners should classify all the health beliefs into two groups: those that are historically rooted in the cultural patterns and lifestyle of the target community, and those that are newly formulated and have only superficial ties with the cultural patterns and lifestyle of the target community.

## Discussion

The implementation of interventions, consistent with PEN-3, should be based on whether health beliefs are long-term and historically rooted in the tradition and culture or more recent, short-term beliefs.

The reinforcement or changing of long-term cultural beliefs should be addressed through health education in the home (home visits) and/or through one-to-one contacts in the community, whereas more recent, non-traditionally entrenched health beliefs can be addressed through the mass media—posters, flyers, radio and television messages, and so on (Airhihenbuwa, 1992; Fuglesang, 1973). It should be noted, however, that although home visits may also be appropriate for changing nonentrenched health beliefs, mass media have not proved effective for changing negative health beliefs that are historically rooted in cultural patterns and lifestyles. Researchers have shown that mass media channels are most effective for increasing knowledge, reinforcing previously held attitudes, and changing behaviors that were recently established or predisposed to change, as opposed to those that are tied to cultural values or are contrary to the attitudes and values expressed in the mass media (Griffiths & Knutson, 1960). In child survival programs, despite the difficulty in organizing an outreach, face-to-face communication channels have been found to be most effective in educating mothers about the use of oral rehydration therapy for persons with diarrhea (Hornik, 1988).

The health educator must understand the rationale behind stated beliefs and practices. To emphasize this point, the Ministry of Health trainers at the workshop discussed above were asked to supervise their village health workers in role plays on health beliefs. This was necessary for them to be able to make appropriate classifications and to select appropriate health education strategies. Moreover, this exercise provided an important demonstration of the ubiquitous nature of some of these beliefs relative to the three dimensions of positive, existential, and negative, and how a given belief may be functional in more than one category, depending on the objective of the health program. For example, when classifying beliefs and practices into positive, existential, and negative beliefs, "Families should have a lot of children because of high child mortality rates" could be classified as a negative belief. However, the health workers in this case classified it as existential, because this belief, which is logical, is a reality for the women living in this community. On the other hand, it could become a positive belief in a vaccination program designed to motivate individuals and families to have fewer children. In another example, the belief that postpartum sexual abstinence prevents semen from mixing with breast milk can be positive in terms of child spacing and allowing a woman ample time to recover following the strain of childbirth. The classification of "immunization as a cause of death" is an example of a recent, non-culturally entrenched belief. This belief was established when some children who had been immunized through EPI later died, after their mothers were told that immunization would prevent their children's deaths. Only face-to-face education has been effective in convincing mothers that immunization may prevent a child from dying from some diseases and that additional preventive measures must be taken to protect children against other illnesses, such as diarrhea and malaria.

Regarding political and institutional factors, another example is helpful. Some health workers had observed that women from certain areas were not taking their children to be immunized. Upon inquiry by an expert trusted by the women, it was discovered that there were cases of children who developed side effects, such as abscesses, from immunization. In addition, the women were asked to pay for treatment of this resultant condition, even though EPI services are free. The health workers recommended to the authorities at the Ministry of Health that they evaluate and try to eliminate any adverse consequences of immunization, and that the ministry should provide treatment free of charge in those cases in which a problem does develop.

When dealing with oral traditions, the focus should not be limited to "how to transform the learner," as is often the case; rather, attention should also be paid to whether or not the interventionist has the requisite skill to transmit knowledge in a culturally appropriate manner. It is important not only to understand the storyteller; it is equally important, if not more so, to understand the dynamics of the story listener. Oral tradition generally is not the heritage solely of the spoken or sung word; it is also the heritage of the ear (Faseke, 1990). Stated differently, people in the oral traditional cultures of several African countries are accustomed to learning by what they hear. Learning by what they see is important to the extent that it is congruent with what they hear and who produces that information. The implication of this pattern of knowledge acquisition for the teacher must be understood and appropriately employed. In other words, if people in an oral traditional culture learn more by listening, the teacher (health educator) should spend more time talking, discussing, and sharing insights than showing pictures or using other audiovisual aids. If talking and sharing ideas constitute the primary mode of learning, health providers (particularly those from other countries) must have adequate competence in oral communication in order to be able to impart knowledge effectively to individuals, families, and the community.

## Lessons From HIV/AIDS Prevention

In response to the need for a culturally appropriate health intervention framework, the PEN-3 method was used to guide the development of an HIV/AIDS education program so as to ensure that cultural beliefs and experiences were considered in exploring and promoting behavior change. The involvement of community members is the key to an adequate assessment of culturally relevant health beliefs and practices and to the planning of appropriate interventions. Jaccard, Turrisi, and Wan (1990) propose that after the high-risk activities of a target population have been identified, two strategies should be considered in attempting to change these behaviors. The first is environmental manipulation, which involves altering or manipulating structural features in the environment that will provide opportunities for the adoption of alternate behaviors. Examples of this strategy include the provision of clean needles to reduce the frequency of needle sharing among intravenous drug users and the provision of condoms to reduce the frequency of unprotected sexual intercourse.

The second strategy is persuasive communication, or the deliberate influencing and modifying of individual beliefs, attitudes, and/or decisions through exposure to information. Source expertise is a critical factor in the use of persuasive communication in AIDS education programs designed for African American communities. Health education staff should include minority members, because these individuals are more knowledgeable than others about the behaviors and values of their communities (Peterson & Bakerman, 1989).

Language, both verbal and nonverbal, is a critical tool of persuasive communication. This must be understood by those attempting to select appropriate interventions for particular racial or ethnic groups. The reinforcement or changing of cultural beliefs should be attempted within the context of the culture's lexicon.

A form of communication prevalent among many African Americans is African American English (AAE), a well-formed and valid linguistic system that encompasses the whole range of language forms used by African Americans throughout the United States (McNair-Knox, 1991). A variation of AAE is African American Vernacular English (AAVE), more commonly called Black Vernacular English or Ebonics, which is associated with the speech of low-income African Americans, particularly young people. The cultural rationale for understanding AAVE is that its use among teens appears to function as an important symbol of peer group solidarity and as a demonstration of pride in African heritage. Vernacular language expression is a window to underlying messages about teen peer identity issues, behavior norms, and reactions to environmental conditions. Efforts to tap into this expression may create a relatively positive and nonthreatening context for communicating with teens, and HIV/AIDS prevention messages must be developed and communicated in a manner that ensures their reception by the members of the groups at greatest risk.

## Conclusion

Several cultural factors can promote or hinder the success of health education programs in developing countries. The future of health education/promotion lies in the ability to centralize these cultural factors within their proper historical and political contexts. For health promotion interventions, particularly in countries of Africa, Latin America, and Asia as well as among ethnic minority populations in industrialized nations, health educators must employ culturally sensitive methods to examine varied health behaviors in terms of positive/beneficial beliefs that must be encouraged, existential/cultural beliefs and practices that do not threaten health, and negative/harmful health practices that should be changed.

In the chapters that follow, I discuss the politics of representation within the context of population subgroups and traditional healing modalities. Examples of the PEN-3 method are presented within the context of each chapter. The examples are meant to generate more discussion, so that cultural dimensions of health can be assessed from positive, existential, and negative perspectives rather than from the sole perspective of negativity. Such negativity has led to the almost automatic coupling of the concept of cultural difference with that of barriers. The PEN-3 examples, therefore, are designed to transform the notion of *cultural barriers* to *cultural dimensions,* wherein barriers are understood as one unfortunate possibility.

# PART II

# Representation and Difference in Health Promotion

# 4

# Health, Healing, and Medicine as Cultural Constructs

> To distinguish the doctor's professional exercise of white magic from his function as engineer (and to spare him the charge of being a quack), the term "placebo" was created. Whenever a sugar pill works because it is given by the doctor, the sugar pill acts as a placebo. A placebo (Latin for "I will please") pleases not only the patient but the administering physician as well.
>
> *Ivan Illich,* Medical Nemesis, *1976*

Traditional healing is perhaps the only health system that is accessible to everyone in Africa. Some 80% of Africans use traditional healing methods (Bannerman, Burton, & Wen-Chieh, 1983). Traditional healing has been sustained over the years partly because it is based in cultural values and norms of the people and partly because it is available, acceptable, and affordable.

Africans' use of traditional remedies to prevent, treat, and cure illness dates back several centuries. In examining health services in Africa, as well as in other parts of the world, health educators and

AUTHOR'S NOTE: This chapter is an expanded and modified version of my chapter, coauthored with Ira E. Harrison, "Traditional Medicine in Africa: Past, Present and Future," in Conrad and Gallagher (Eds.), *Health and Health Care in Developing Countries.* (pp. 122-134). Copyright © 1993 by Temple University Press. Used by permission.

designers of health promotion programs must consider the cultural framework carefully in order to understand how indigenous peoples view sickness, disease, and appropriate treatment methods (Airhihenbuwa, 1990-1991; Harvey, 1988).

Researchers who study health practices and beliefs are now cognizant of the fact that patients and clients who seek prevention or cure for illness or disease do so in a variety of ways, and that prevention and cure are sought from a variety of sources (Dennis, 1985). Moreover, it is now well understood that the sources of prevention and cure of particular problems are determined to a great extent by the clients' sociocultural and religious backgrounds (Airhihenbuwa, 1987; Holzer, 1973). Because Africa's cultural evolution has often been misrepresented, it is no surprise that its healing modalities have been victims of allopathic hegemony. In Africa, the harsh experiences and upheavals of the slave trade, colonialism, and neocolonialism precluded the pattern of development experienced in the West. Similarly, the evolution of traditional medicine in African countries is different from that of countries that were not colonized, such as China.

In all forms of traditional healing, religion and shared cultural values and beliefs are at the core of preventive and curative health practices. Religion, magic, and superstition and their resulting practices (e.g., traditional medicine) are all based on rationality. Such rationality is best understood in its traditional (emic) context rather than through a Western (etic) paradigm, hence the popular utilization of traditional medicine in developing countries. An etic approach is one that focuses on universal traits regardless of culture, whereas an emic approach focuses on cultural differences (Pike, 1954, cited in Pedersen, Draguns, Conner, & Trimble, 1981; see also Kegley & Saviers, 1983). However, it is useful for health educators to explore the possibilities offered by both systems of medicine, so that Africans can utilize the most effective health care services for different conditions and under differing circumstances.

## Reappraisal of Traditional Health Care

It is a commonly and easily observed fact that even the most "detribalized" and "modernized" Christians, scholars, scientists, and entrepreneurs among the African bourgeoisie today still consult African divinities, diviners, and healers when their health or other affairs are in serious trouble. Many have been known to sneak away from their church pews, discard their three-piece suits, steal away by night to some healer in his forest shrine, and carry out all manner of ritual sacrifices when these are demanded. In fact, even among those with Ph.D.s, D.Sc.s, LL.D.s, and other assorted strings of Western bourgeois academic degrees, the going attitude is still that Western medicines and the Western Christian God are fine in their place, but when things get tough, one runs back to one's roots and ancestral ways (Chinweizu, Jemie, & Madubuike, 1983, p. 21).

The existence or absence of a large corpus of literature on a country's traditional medicine tends to depend on whether or not the country is colonized and the extent to which the colonizers have outlawed the practice and consequently the documentation of traditional medicine. In the nineteenth century and most of the twentieth, Europeans were concerned with colonization, exploitation, and commerce. Janzen (1974-1975), in a discussion of Belgian colonial policy in the Congo, notes that "indigenous therapeutic practices were never mentioned within colonial manuals or laws. These laws sought only to establish European-modelled institutions regardless of what may have pre- or co-existed in African society" (p. 109). Ralph Schram's *A History of Nigerian Health Services* (1971) never mentions the traditional healers who were serving the people prior to the colonizing exercises of the British (cited in Harrison, 1984).

During the early part of the twentieth century, there was a shift of emphasis from conquest of Africans, Asians, Latin Americans, and Oceanic peoples to control and co-optation of these peoples. This shift in emphasis was aimed at the maintenance of law, order, and economic growth. Thus non-Western beliefs and values were ignored. The medical beliefs and practices of most non-European peoples were considered primitive, savage, and barbaric; they were considered not medicine, but magic, religion, or witchcraft (Seijas, 1975). As a result, laws were promulgated to criminalize the practice of traditional medicine.

A few decades later, Bronislaw Malinowski (1954) and A. R. Radcliffe-Brown (1952) learned that religious rites, beliefs, and practices served to maintain order in society and to regulate individual and group sentiment and behavior. Religious rites have a specific social function, namely, to regulate, maintain, and transmit from one generation to another the sentiments on which the constitution of the society depends. "Generally speaking, religious ceremonies take believers away from the mundane affairs of life, sometimes by presenting exhilarating experiences" (Harvey, 1988, p. 103). Religion is critical to an understanding of the spiritual dimension of health, which in turn is pivotal to the maintenance of the psychosocial dimension of health. In other words, there is more to health care than medical care. Health care delivery systems do not exist in and of themselves, but as parts of larger sociocultural wholes. Health care systems comprise a set of resources that may serve nonmedical as well as medical goals.

A reassessment of the disease-focused approach to health care has led many social and behavioral scientists to adopt a social action approach to health care delivery, particularly in Southern countries. This means that the views of the community (the emic perspective) are now believed to be as important as, if not more important than, "scientific" views (etic perspectives). Medical and health beliefs and practices that had in the past been deemed superstitions are being reassessed and given fresh interpretations. These beliefs constitute symbolic representations of various realities, many of which are non-Western. Maladies resulting from hot-cold imbalance, the dislocation of internal organs, impure blood, unclean air, moral transgression, interpersonal struggle, and humans' relation to the spirit world are now seen as different manifestations of some general reality. When people define physical or emotional symptoms within a traditional taxonomy, they are likely to seek help in the traditional health care system. Thus, as Nigerian health education specialist Z. A. Ademuwagun (1974-1975) indicates, Nigerians in the Ibarapa district of Oyo state use traditional healers for excessive worry, sleeplessness, malaria, yellow fever, and snakebite. T. A. Lambo (1978), retired deputy director general of the World Health Organization (WHO), faults the Western medical practitioner as being "invariably preoccupied with immediate natural causes, almost to the exclusion of the causal relations between conflicts and irregularities in the field of social relations on the one hand and disease or misfortune on the other." Traditional healers generally became a focus of research because they were thought to have knowledge about herbal concoctions that may be useful in treating such health problems as hypertension, diabetes, and other chronic diseases that Westerners have found difficult if not impossible to cure (Harrison, 1974).

## Traditional Healing Concepts

The belief that a state of balance exists within the individual on the one hand and between the individual and the environment on the other is a concept that is true for all traditional healing modalities worldwide. How this concept is operationalized varies among cultures and hence among different traditional healing systems. African traditional medicine seeks to secure and maintain a balance among the individual, elements of nature, and the heavenly bodies. Within the individual, a balance is maintained among organic disorders, physiological disorders, and social conflicts. This balanced state is, in turn, balanced with elements of nature—earth, fire, water, air, and metal. Finally, balance is sought with the heavenly bodies—the sun, moon, and stars.

Organic and physiological disorders are concepts that are familiar to allopathic medicine. Social conflict is also a familiar allopathic concept in understanding psychological disorders. Expressions such as "He gets under my skin" and "She makes me sick" are examples of manifestations of social conflicts. In the African traditional healing context, an understanding of social conflict is pivotal to curing a person who has become ill. This is where the healer deals with the *ultimate* cause of an illness: who or what caused it, and why. The *proximate* cause, or specific etiology, tells only how it happened, not why it happened. For people who believe in this concept of disease nosology, knowledge of germ theory is useful only for explaining the medium through which health problems manifest themselves.

Ultimately, the origin of the disease or malady must be explained and dealt with. The body, mind, and environment must function in harmony for the individual to experience optimum health. In fact, in homeopathy, disease symptoms are considered good indications of the body's attempt to heal itself. For example, shivering in cold weather is the body's attempt to generate more heat in order to increase the core temperature of the body, and one should potentiate the shivering process rather than stop it; high fever is the body's attempt to make the environment uncomfortable for germs; and the cold and clammy skin of a person in shock is the result of the smaller blood vessels' diverting blood to the vital organs for the person's survival. The human body's ability to regulate itself naturally, as well as to synchronize the functions of its various parts to maintain a state of balance and harmony, is a basic principle of traditional medicine. It is this natural mechanism for dealing with states of balance and imbalance that traditional healers have always understood and attempted to maintain.

Traditional medicine is a desirable part of a nation's formal health care system, particularly in rural areas. Some 70% of the Western-trained doctors in Nigeria live in six cities (Benin, Enugu, Ibadan, Ife, Lagos, and Zaria) (Osuntokun, 1975), and most of the country's rural population relies solely on traditional practitioners to care for their health needs (Oyebola, 1986). Therefore, it behooves health professionals to examine the strengths and weaknesses of traditional medicine, so that they can promote its strengths and discourage its weaknesses for the benefit of the people who believe in it and use it.

Traditional medicine has paralleled the practice of Western allopathic medicine in a number of ways. In 1879, Robert Felkin, a British medical missionary traveling in Baganda (modern-day Uganda), reported a high level of medical and health practice. He saw the successful performance of cesarean sections, with antiseptic techniques, by a native surgical team. He also saw experiments devised to discover a cure for a local epidemic (J. N. P. Davis, 1959). Although Felkin witnessed this only two years after Joseph Lister advocated antisepsis use in surgery in London, it was clear to Felkin that the team's "surgical technique" and "public health experiments" were a part of the tradition of the Baganda. This suggests that the use of antisepsis by the traditional healers of Baganda predates its use by allopathic surgeons.

Other contributions made by traditional healers to health care delivery include the discovery of many herbal remedies, including *Rauwolfia serpentina,* a medicinal plant known as snakeroot, whose active ingredient, reserpine, is used today as a tranquilizer and hypotensive agent (Basch, 1990); *Erythropleum guineense,* identified from the bark of the sasswood tree, a powerful laxative substance (Foster, 1963); and *Periwinkle vinca rosea,* an herb containing insulin, which is used in the treatment of diabetes mellitus (Foster, 1963; Teller, 1968).

In addition to their contributions in the use of medicinal plants, traditional healers have been very successful in treating psychosomatic disorders. Lambo (1961) provides an example of healers' (*babalawos* of Nigeria) ingenuity:

> A toad is tied to the penis of the bed wetter. If the child urinates, the heat from the urine wakes up the toad who then begins to croak. The croaking of the toad wakes up the child. The similarity of this device to the modern anuretic machine is evident. The modern anuretic machine delivers a shock to the bed wetter on urinating. Behaviorally speaking, the electric shock and the croaking of the toad function as negative reinforcers.

Another example was shared by a British-trained physician from Mauritius who attended a lecture I gave on traditional medicine in June 1991 as part of the Boston University School of Public Health summer certificate program titled Health Care in Developing Countries. He recounted the story of a Nigerian soccer player who had suffered a compound leg fracture in the 1970s and was healed by a traditional bonesetter. When the limb healed, however, it was shorter than the uninjured limb, such that the patient was left with a limp. The patient went back to the traditional healer to seek a solution, and was instructed as follows: He was to ask a friend or relative to go to the river with him and tie him up in the part of the river with the heaviest wave for one hour every day. At the end of six months, the patient's broken leg was back to its normal length—the strength of the river's current had realigned the bone properly. This approach was of course very different from the one that would have been taken in an allopathic system, in which the bone would have been rebroken in a hospital and reset. Although it would be naive to suggest that traditional medicine is a panacea for the health problems of Africans, it certainly has the proven potential to improve the health care delivery system significantly for many people.

An understanding of the function of traditional medicine in any culture must begin with an understanding of the culture and its history. This is a challenge for behavioral and social scientists who have an interest in solving the health problems of developing countries. As a result of the renewed interest in traditional medicine, partly because of the primary health care movement and more recently the child survival revolution, the integration concept is now in vogue. Even given the problems that have been identified in the integration of traditional medicine with allopathic approaches (Pillsbury, 1982), international donor agencies concerned with primary health care, child survival, and safe motherhood have all displayed interest in such integration in their programs. However, often these agencies view the potential contributions of traditional medicine as very limited. On the strength of their economic resources, such agencies have dominated health policy and practices in the Third World since World War II (Justice, 1987). Along with their influence and funding resources have come policy guidelines and priorities that have always promoted allopathic hegemony.

Major difficulties with government policy arise from perceptions and definitions of traditional medicine. Murray Last (1986) observes:

> Though within most nations there are usually a large number of medical sub-cultures, each with its own characteristics and structure, policy-makers often have in mind apparently a single, paradigmatic culture from which they generalize about "traditional medicine." Inevitably such stereotypes are likely to reflect political conditions—as of course happened under colonial rule when traditional healers were categorized as "witches." (p. 4)

## Issues of Integration

Failure to historicize traditional healing has resulted in misguided efforts by allopaths, albeit with sincere intentions, to address the formalization of traditional healing within the health care system. Historically, traditional healers were specialists at a time when allopaths were generalists. Healers specialized in diagnostics, maternal and child care, bonesetting, and so on. The earliest attempts by governments to legitimate and confirm traditional healers encountered difficulties when physicians, who were generalists, proposed to traditional healers, who were specialists, that they should all come together under one umbrella as traditional healers. The impetus for such unification was to standardize traditional practice rather than for political and social leverage, as in the case of allopaths. Because the bonesetters could never understand the wisdom of a forced marriage with maternal and child health specialists (even though a few might specialize in both), unification never materialized. In cases in which unification has occurred today, it is for the same reason as Western allopathic unification—political leverage within a society. It should be noted, however, that approaches to specialization have changed for both traditional healers and allopaths. Whereas physicians now train to become specialists, traditional healers train to become generalists. These transitions have been fueled by the desire to maximize economic leverage.

Physicians continue to be suspicious of traditional healers because, they assert, healers blame their patients when the patients fail to recover. In their defense of standardization, physicians claim to assume responsibility for the deaths of patients by coming together with their colleagues (in professional standards reviews) and discussing how to learn from mistakes so as not to repeat them. Physicians see this not as professional secrecy, but simply as professionalism. However, when asked whether physicians would be satisfied with traditional healers' "professionalism" if healers were to meet regularly to discuss the outcome of fatal cases, physicians respond with a resounding no.

Thus, as perceived by physicians, professional responsibility comprises differing values, expectations, and interpretations for physicians and traditional healers. Few, if any, physicians will actually go to the family of a deceased patient to take responsibility for the death, even though that is what they expect of traditional healers. Moreover, many physicians fail to see that suggesting to the family of a patient who has just undergone an operation that "it is now up to the patient" or that "the patient's will to live is very important at this time" is a form of holding the patient personally responsible for his or her recovery and thus blaming the patient if he or she dies.

Physicians who insist that allopathic medicine is purely scientific, objective, and measurable are strongly opposed to keeping score cards that might compare their professional skills with those of their peers, on the grounds that there are other factors that make medicine less objective and measurable, and perhaps less scientific. Yet physicians accuse healers of being unscientific and insist that healers be subject to individual objective and scientific evaluation—the very measures of professional performance to which they are strongly opposed for themselves.

It seems quite apparent that in medicine there are certain levels of nonscientific, subjective, and perhaps even "magical" practices. The "scientific" aspects and the "human aspects" jointly potentiate the possibilities of healing. Illich aptly notes this invoking of magic in allopathic practices in the epigraph that opens this chapter. The belief in magic within the Western "scientific framework" is not exclusive to medicine. Perhaps the most revealing of Western superstitions is the fact that many modern, shiny, glass-and-steel skyscrapers, financed, built, owned, managed, and occupied by the cream of Western bourgeoisie, have no thirteenth floors. Of course, the thirteenth floors are simply numbered 14 to deceive the witches, ghosts, and other evil spirits (Chinweizu et al., 1983, p. 22)!

In 1977, the Thirtieth World Health Assembly adopted a resolution (WHA 30.49) urging governments to give "adequate importance to the utilization of their traditional systems of medicine, with appropriate regulations" (Akerele, 1984, p. 77). This became the stimulus that galvanized the World Health Organization to launch the global promotion of traditional medicine. It has been estimated that 80% or more of the world's rural population relies mainly on traditional medicines for health care needs (Bannerman et al., 1983). Three major recommendations have been made concerning (a) evaluation of traditional healing practices, (b) incorporation of traditional medicine as part of national health care systems, and (c) provision of training for traditional healers. To accomplish this goal, attempts have been made in different countries to find common ground for traditional medicine and allopathic medicine. The struggle to locate this common ground has led many to advocate for the integration of these two kinds of care systems. Such integration has been promoted by many respected organizations, including WHO and UNICEF, and scholars such as Bannerman et al. (1983), Lambo (1978), Akerele (1984), Pillsbury (1982), Maclean and Bannerman (1982), and Newman and Bhatia (1973).

Unfortunately, the implementation of integration has been based on a "donor-deficit model" for the traditional healers. The guiding belief is that traditional healers can be trained to "modernize" their healing practices by having allopathic professionals teach them what they do not know (that is, healers are assessed from a deficit model). In the process, allopaths find out what traditional healers know, so that their knowledge can be improved when applied to allopathic practice (healers become donors). The assumption is usually made that the healer, who supposedly needs some training, can make little or no contribution to improving the knowledge and practice of the allopath.

In discussions about the integration of traditional and allopathic health services, seldom has the traditional healer been viewed as a health provider with adequate or superior knowledge in certain aspects of health care that will be of benefit to the allopathic provider (physician) in a training session. The sources of traditional healers' concoctions and pharmacopoeia, however, are eagerly, even exploitatively, sought (Harrison & Cosminsky, 1976). Though deficient in some areas, traditional healers could be donors in other areas. Instead of receiving proper and due recognition for the areas in which they are known to be efficient and effective, healers are encouraged to surrender their herbal lore for the advancement of science.

Such mistakes in professional judgment do not end with allopathic physicians. Some behavioral and social scientists who believe in aspirin yet cannot explain how it relieves pain have demanded that traditional healers explain their medications before these scientists consider the medications valid, even though they are used for the same reason as aspirin—a strong belief in its healing power. This kind of inconsistent and one-sided judgment has led to reluctance and suspicion on the part of traditional health care providers. Instead of integration or cooperation based on mutual trust, respect, and collaboration, in most cases the outcomes are distrust and suspicion.

As one explores the concept of integration further, three problems become evident. First, as stated above, the healer is seen as one who needs to be trained but who has nothing to contribute to training the allopath. Second, a conflict exists between didactic learning, which is how allopaths are trained, and experiential learning, which is how traditional healers are trained. Third, there is a lack of systematic protection of ownership of orally transmitted information, which is a vital form of intellectual and creative property in traditional medicine.

Integration has been more successful in the area of childbirth practices than in other areas of traditional medicine (Pillsbury, 1982). This success has often been attributed to traditional birth attendants' not posing any serious competition to physicians in terms of their professional status, power, and resources (Green, 1988). In other cases of integration, governments have attempted to incorporate traditional healers into modern sector projects or programs (Pillsbury, 1982). These attempts almost always involve some kind of training for the healers to upgrade their knowledge. Unfortunately, the healers often receive training in the most basic and mundane tasks, such as mixing oral rehydration solutions, even though the healers would like to learn how to give injections and read X rays (Green, 1988).

A training session designed for integration should be one in which both allopathic providers (particularly physicians) and traditional healers are trainers and trainees, because both have information to contribute and to gain. Integration should mean the involvement of healers in the planning, implementation, and evaluation of health services delivery in order to foster cooperation and participation. This does not necessarily mean moving the traditional healer to a hospital setting, any more than it should mean moving the physician to the healer's practice setting. Integration, for example, may mean appropriate referral from a physician to a bonesetter for fractures, as well as referral from an herbalist to an internist for appendicitis.

The second problem with integration is that of the often ignored differences between allopathic and traditional healers in methods of knowledge acquisition, as applied to proposed training programs. Paramount among these are differences in perceptions of reality. Formal, didactic teaching is not usefully applied to traditional healing practice, in which learning in the apprenticeship mode (experiential learning) is more appropriate and culturally customary (Jordan, 1989). This is particularly true of the several training programs developed to "upgrade" the knowledge and skills of traditional birth attendants—the ubiquitous, taken-for-granted midwives (Maclean & Bannerman, 1982, p. 1815).

The third problem with integration is that physicians have arrogantly requested that traditional healers share their knowledge about their treatments and medicines without setting up any systematic process to guarantee ownership of the information that is revealed. In Western culture, the protection of information, inventions, and discoveries and their revelation is guaranteed under copyright and patent laws. In a U.N. debate over how Southern nations are to be rewarded for contributions to plant species, Henry Shands, a U.S. delegate, argued that without a strong patent law there is no incentive for people to investigate the possible superior medicinal properties of plant species (Simons, 1989).

Although patent and copyright laws are not customary in oral tradition, revelation of information within this context has always been protected. One method of such protection has been for healers to reveal information only to one or two protégés. Thus open, widespread revelation is an allopathic phenomenon and should carry with it the protection and rewards that go with it or, alternatively, a culturally appropriate modified version. When traditional healers possess the knowledge to discover, create, and use compounds of superior medicinal properties, such information should not be shared with others in the absence of some system guaranteeing that the original sources of such information or medication are protected and/or appropriately rewarded for its revelation. Although healers may not articulate such a right, it is a basic human desire to receive the comfort and protection of these fundamental principles regarding information sharing and proprietorship, regardless of the pattern of knowledge acquisition.

Such protection and rights of ownership are paramount in promoting open information sharing and true reciprocity between and among health providers and policy makers. The resistance of physicians to sharing information with traditional healers could be considered an example of such protection. It should, however, be noted that such reluctance about integration is not unique to physicians. It is also true of medical anthropologists, medical sociologists, health educators, and other public health professionals. However, the stakes are much higher for the public when healers, both allopathic and traditional, do not cooperate with each other to maximize health coverage for the people so that the public might benefit from the best of both worlds.

International health professionals will have a better appreciation of international health problems if they understand that treatment modalities, like diseases and disease patterns, are intricately tied to beliefs and values within cultures. As long as Africans successfully seek treatment from both allopathic and traditional healers, it is prudent to strive for mutual collaboration based on respect and trust between the two types of health providers. Perhaps the word should be *cooperation* instead of *integration.* The latter tends to conjure up resistance among those who interpret this process as an encroachment on their territory. This has been my experience during workshops and lectures on traditional medicine. If the PEN-3 method is used, beliefs and perceptions can be grouped into positive, existential, and negative domains, so that a complete and balanced view on a given modality can be obtained.

## Implications for National Health Policy

An important factor contributing to successful national health policy in Southern countries is clear definition of the healing modalities. Such a definition should involve people from both allopathic and traditional healing systems. As Last (1986) advocates, traditional healers ought to organize themselves and seek professional status, in order not only to survive but to get their share of government support. Integration, registration, and professionalization, however, may be possible only after a period of official government recognition. Such recognition may take various forms, at various levels, in various contexts (Harrison, 1984). By *recognition,* I mean an array of relationships among traditional healers, government officials, and medical personnel that may range from private meetings to licensure. Healers, traditional or modern, are human and therefore may interact and exchange information as family members, friends, and professionals.

Policy makers should decide on communities' unmet health needs and then involve social and behavioral scientists, as well as community members, in health program planning, implementation, and evaluation. The community thus helps to define acceptable healing practices based on indigenous reasoning, which may be inexplicable in the Western context. Cultural diversity among peoples of different nations and the impact of such diversity on program replicability cannot be overemphasized. Community involvement is one strategy for acknowledging the impact of culture on a national health system. This is often realized when the individuals, families, and communities for whom a program is intended, as well as service providers (traditional healers), have the opportunity to be a part of the team that defines the health problems to be targeted and formulates their solution through design of a particular health program. Sensitivity to traditional customs and social norms, and thus cultural appropriateness of a program, is ensured through the participation of community members.

Allopathic health providers can learn from traditional healers, just as traditional healers can learn from allopathic practitioners. Understanding the components of a system of healing is critical to the ability to influence the health behavior of those who subscribe to that system. Consequently, health educators should learn to be more humble about their profession and programs and should strive to become more understanding of others (Torrey, 1972). Some allopathic physicians have already started to utilize what they have learned from traditional healers. Some now place an amulet around a child's neck in order to ensure that the child returns for a follow-up visit, so the physician can maintain continuity of care until the patient is cured. Reciprocally, some traditional healers now send their fracture patients to have their bones X-rayed in a hospital. In child survival programs, the traditional wearing of beads around a child's wrist is being used for growth monitoring. Thus there is already some level of cooperation.

## Conclusion

One of the key primary health care providers in most Southern countries is the traditional healer. Because traditional medicine is based on cultural and traditional values, it is important for health educators to affirm and legitimate this modality within the formal health care system. Ignoring traditional medicine is tantamount to ignoring the cultural impact of health and disease in these societies. After all, one cannot sincerely address health care delivery in Africa without giving adequate coverage to traditional medicine. Social and behavioral scientists who are interested in health care delivery in Southern nations should devote adequate time to an exploration of the past, present, and future contributions of traditional healers to health care delivery in these countries. This was done, for example, when the WHO Global Programme on AIDS and Traditional Medicine Programme convened an informal consultation in Geneva in February 1989 to review the status of research and services in traditional medicine as applied to HIV infection and AIDS (World Health Organization, 1989).

Social and behavioral health scientists must be willing to experiment with various forms, at different levels, and with definitive contexts in order to establish and promote proper communication with traditional and allopathic health providers. Communication and cooperation must prevail if there is to be an optimal working relationship between these forms of health services. Therefore, social and behavioral scientists have critical roles to play in improving global health care policies and systems, and it is vital that they work with traditional healers to ensure the provision of adequate health care systems in Southern nations. Such systems will ensure that Africans have available, accessible, acceptable, and affordable health services and will allow all Africans to benefit from the best of both worlds (Akerele, 1986).

# 5

# African Women's Health and the Confluence of Patriarchal and Western Hegemonies

> The true worth of a race must be measured by the character of its womanhood.
>
> *Mary McLeod Bethune, "A Century of Progress of Negro Women," 1933*

Whereas in one culture an individual's opportunities to make decisions that ultimately shape his or her destiny may rest with the person's level of independence in both the family and society, in other cultures it is an individual's level of autonomy that determines such decision-making ability. Autonomy is often confused with independence, especially when discussion focuses, cross-culturally, on the issue of social and economic freedom for women. Autonomy does not necessarily require that one be independent of one's family or partner, as long as one's role and contribution in society are duly recognized and valued economically, culturally, and socially. The issues of autonomy and independence undergird the differences in how Western women and African women view the plight of women in general.

One of the issues related to the role of men in women's oppression is the economic valuation of women's contribution to family stability and growth. When it is a question of serving their own interests, men conceive of work only in terms of payment, but when it is a question of valorizing the rights of women, they find it absurd that women demand to be paid for their services (needless to say, the housewife works even if she is helped by a maid, just as men in the workplace give to their subordinates all the burdensome tasks) and appeal to the duties of love. Thus the ambiguity of giving and of duty is manipulated at will by men according to the circumstances (Minh-ha, 1991).

African women are no different from Western women in terms of working long hours and receiving few or no remunerative and/or social supports and rewards commensurate with their labor. Having to work under these conditions, women naturally have the need and desire to seek efficient and effective ways to use available human and material resources to reduce their workload and enjoy some leisure time during the day. The differences between African and Western women in general lie in the opportunities and liberty they have to use such resources (e.g., human resources such as children or material resources such as domestic technology) as well as to manage the environment (such as family expectations) to achieve life's goals. For example, many African women do not have at their disposal domestic appliances, such as machines for pounding *fufu* or *cassava* or individual and/or accessible neighborhood washing machines and dryers, which could relieve them of some of the burden of their endless, arduous tasks. Yet men can always purchase motorized vehicles (as opposed, for example, to bicycles) for transportation and can even afford luxury items such as stereos, televisions, and VCRs. In fact, when Yam Poundo (a machine for pounding yam) became available at a reasonable price (less than the price of an average stereo) in Nigeria in the early 1980s, many men who could afford one would not buy one for their wives because they believed that the machine did not pound yam as smoothly as could a woman using mortar and pestle. Needless to say, some of their wives agreed. This seeming complicity of the wives can be seen as the propagation of values internalized over time, even though such values may not serve one's interest. However, it should be noted that there will always be initial skepticism in adopting a new product, particularly when it challenges the perceived usefulness of traditional practice.

Those men who bought and encouraged their wives to use the machine did so after they found out that the pounded yam they ate in their favorite restaurants was made in such machines. Thus, even when the new technology was finally adopted, it was not adopted because of its benefits in time effectiveness and efficiency for wives, but because husbands realized that it would not compromise their interest (the taste of the yam). This is an attempt not to demonize maleness, but rather to problematize the way in which patriarchal domination is nurtured and reinforced even by men who may believe in the struggle for gender equality.

Where the Western woman complains of being doubly oppressed, the Black woman of Africa suffers threefold oppression: patriarchal domination by virtue of her sex, capitalist exploitation by virtue of her class, and appropriation of her country by colonial or neocolonial powers by virtue of her race (Thiam, 1986). The historical terrain of oppression perpetuated by men on women has tended to parallel the patterns of cultures that otherwise embody totally different values and meanings. Such a seemingly synchronized time line among and between different cultures in constructing and executing patriarchal hegemony is captured by Achebe (1987):

> The original oppression of Woman was based on crude denigration. They caused Man to fall. So she became a scapegoat. No, not a scapegoat which might be blameless but a culprit richly deserving of whatever suffering Man chose thereafter to heap on her. That is Woman in the Book of Genesis. Out here, our ancestors, without the benefit of hearing about the Old Testament, made the very same story differing only in local colour. At first the Sky was very close to the Earth. But every evening Woman cut off a piece of the Sky to put in her soup pot or, as in another version, she repeatedly banged the top end of her pestle carelessly against the Sky whenever she pounded the millet or, as in yet another rendering—so prodigious is Man's inventiveness—she wiped her kitchen hands on the Sky's face. Whatever the detail of Woman's provocation, the Sky finally moved away in anger, and God with it. Well, that kind of candid chauvinism might be OK for the rugged taste of the Old Testament. The New Testament required a more enlightened, more refined, more loving even, strategy—ostensibly, that is. So the idea came to Man to turn his spouse into the very Mother of God, to pick her up from right under his foot where she'd been since Creation and carry her reverently to a nice,

> corner pedestal. Up there, her feet completely off the ground, she will be just as irrelevant to the practical decisions of running the world as she was in her bad old days. The only difference is that now Man will suffer no guilt feelings; he can sit back and congratulate himself on his generosity and gentlemanliness. Meanwhile our ancestors out here, unaware of the New Testament, were working out independently a parallel subterfuge of their own. *Nneka,* they said. Mother is supreme. Let us keep her in reserve until the ultimate crisis arrives and the waist is broken and hung over the fire, and the palm bears its fruit at the tail of its leaf. Then, as the world crashes around Man's ears, Woman in her supremacy will descend and sweep the shards together. (p. 89)

The gender inequity in African culture is a process that begins in the family and is perpetuated through cultural values and beliefs and institutionally reinforced throughout society. For example, the father who has three sons and three daughters but only enough resources to provide a solid foundation for the future well-being and social and economic independence (e.g., education) for four of his children may choose to do so for all three sons, no matter their birth order, and then choose one "lucky" daughter. Already the boys are ahead, thus marking the beginning of their privileged position. Everything else that follows serves only to perpetuate the foundation that has been established in the family. In the traditional African philosophy, knowledge obtained through Western formal education is a power that should be reserved only for males, who will inherit the land, thus placing women at great disadvantage (Njoku, 1980). Even when equal foundations are established for all of a family's children, regardless of sex, landownership issues remain a measure of inequality between men and women. The point here is not to demonize maleness and romanticize femaleness, but to illustrate the historical genealogy of the nature of patriarchal domination in many African cultures. This is the only way to address the dismantling of the tools of women's oppression. Such dismantling will require the collective effort of men and women. The involvement of men is critical in the promotion of equity through, among other things, the elimination of different forms of oppression of women. This is why women of African descent differ from White feminists in the nature of women's emancipatory projects. As bell hooks (1993) has stated, "I believe that men must be part of the feminist movement, and they must feel that they have a major role to play in the eradication of sexism. The term 'women's movement' reproduces the notion that somehow feminism is this plantation that only women should labor on" (p. 37).[1]

Women in general suffer oppression in a male-constructed world, but the women of Black Africa suffer additionally from being left out of women's struggle by White women. Most analysts who have evaluated the oppression of women in Africa have tended to view women only in the role of wife. White feminists, for the most part, do not engage in a dialogue on the contradictions that constitute and shape the role of Black women in a family context, as sisters, aunts, or daughters (Amos & Parmar, 1984). African woman's agency is invoked as "daughter" and "sister," yet these dimensions tend to be missing in attempts, particularly by Westerners, to gauge the praxis of women's rights in African countries. What is often highlighted is female circumcision or mutilation, a practice that is opposed by many Africans, particularly feminists/womanists, as they are better able to situate such oppositional projects within the cultural framework under which this practice is promoted. Amos and Parmar (1984) note: "Many White feminists have argued that as feminists they find it very difficult to accept arranged marriages which they see as reactionary. Our argument is that it is not up to them to accept or reject arranged marriages but up to us to challenge, accept, or reform, depending on our various perspectives, on our own terms and in our own culturally specific ways" (p. 15). Dawit and Mekuria (1993) assert:

> A media campaign in the West will not stop genital mutilation. Westerners and those of us living in the West who wish to work on this issue must forge partnerships with the hundreds of African women on the continent who are working to eradicate the practice. Neither Alice Walker nor any of us here can speak for them; but if we have the power and the resources, we can create the room for them to speak, and to speak with us. (p. A27)[2]

Some observers have pointed out that African feminists have not imposed facial surgery (or is it facial mutilation?) on Western feminists as a cultural project. Cosmetic surgery for beauty enhancement is tied to Western normative standards of beauty. This standard, to a large extent, is dictated by male preferences and expectations of beauty. For example, breast augmentation is clearly a glaring case of female internalization of the male gaze. Some might argue that both breast augmentation and facial mutilation are voluntary. However, there is nothing voluntary about individual actions that are taken to fulfill societal expectations, whether such expectations are metaphysically enforced by the individual or directly promoted and implemented by the community. To suggest that facial surgery/mutilation is voluntary, as opposed to circumcision/genital mutilation, is to believe naively that societal forces do not significantly shape human behavior. One can only imagine the number of people who would undergo facial, breast, or other bodily transformation/mutilation if such services were free or inexpensive. Excision and infibulation are deeply rooted in the societies in which they are practiced, which is why protests against these practices by young women are often met with strong resistance on the part of older women (Thiam, 1986).

Pedagogical projects designed to subvert violence against women must historicize such violence within the context of culture and then affirm the efforts of feminists/womanists in that culture to subvert the violence, so that they can serve as legitimate voices and representation for the oppressed. It is important to note that passive resistance is a recognized and legitimate strategy that has been used effectively by the oppressed to subvert oppression. In other words, the oppressed have always believed that when one thing stands, another thing must stand beside it. The oppressed are not always powerless in the grassroots enterprise, as the notion of development participation would suggest. As Rahnema (1992) notes:

> Theirs is a different power which is not always perceived as such, and cannot be actualized in the same manner, yet it is very real in many ways. It is constituted by the thousands of centres and informal networks of resistance which ordinary people put up, often quietly, against the prevailing power apparatuses. Amongst others, it manifests itself in the reality of "tax payers cheating the state, young people evading conscription, farmers accepting subsidies or equipment from development projects and diverting them to their own ends, technicians or repairmen working without permits or licenses, government paid teachers using the classroom to denounce government abuses of power." (p. 123)

Although American and European feminists can represent a voice for oppressed women in other societies, if they try to do so without affirming the work of their comrades in those societies, their work becomes a form of White female hegemony as well as cultural chauvinism. Such cultural chauvinism is the basis of the economic reductionism of Third World Women as found in the literature on women in development. Mohanty (1991b) notes: "The best examples of universalization on the basis of economic reductionism can be found in the liberal 'Women in Development' literature. Proponents of this school seek to examine the effect of development on third world women, sometimes from self-designated feminist perspectives" (p. 63). One avenue where African women are constantly spoken for by their Western counterparts is through the ubiquitous nongovernmental organizations (NGOs).

> Fertility issues and third world women's incorporation into multinational factory employment are identified as two of the most significant aspects of "women's worlds" in third world countries. While such descriptive information is useful and necessary, these presumably "objective" indicators by no means exhaust the meaning of women's day-to-day lives. The everyday, fluid, fundamentally historical and dynamic nature of the lives of third world women is here collapsed into a few frozen "indicators" of their well-being. (Mohanty, 1991a, p. 6)

A number of the Western-based NGOs that are involved in health and development projects in African countries regularly deliberate over the most effective and efficient methods of promoting economic independence among women. One recommendation has been to train more women in income-generating activities for the sustainability of such projects as the child survival programs. "Gardening" is an occupation often recommended as suitable for women, but the nature of work suggests that what is actually being recommended is farming. *Gardening* seems to be a more acceptable term because it romanticizes the labor involved. It suggests that the work is pleasurable and not as rigorous as farming. On the other hand, one cannot help but wonder if middle-class professionals, particularly women, are weary of being accused of encouraging their "sisters" to engage in farming. Whatever the reasons for recommending gardening, it is clear that if such activity were being recommended for men, it would be called farming. Breast-feeding is another example of a practice that can be learned and promoted from within the culture, yet many NGOs now believe they have the requisite knowledge to train African women in how to breast-feed. There is little interest in challenging, for example, the promotion of infant formulas in these countries by Western-based corporations—a practice that has led to the abandonment of breast-feeding by some women for what is unfortunately believed to be a superior form of infant feeding. The NGOs that engage in teaching breast-feeding have made the assumption that if women from Southern nations do not breast-feed their babies, it is because they do not know how.

There are physiological events that occur only in womanhood (i.e., menstruation and menopause) that have been used by different cultures to fault women for the gender gap that has been established and perpetuated by men. Most cultures now embrace the medicalization of menstruation and menopause, such that the onsets of these natural events are marked by negativity. Both physical and emotional isolation and ostracism are commonly associated with the experiences of menstruating or menopausal women. Both of these events may be viewed as part of natural aging processes, but societal (Western medical) responses tend to suggest that many still believe they are pathologic. Very little emphasis is placed on preparing young girls for menarche, and because of the negativity associated with and the medicalization of menopause, there is little interest in understanding how women in traditional cultures experience this life stage. W. Kamau (personal communication, 1993) interviewed some elderly Kenyan women and found that traditional women never experienced any of the typically expected psychomedical manifestations, such as hot flashes, irritability, and depression. Whether or not this is representative of the experiences of most women in Kenya and other African countries, it is clear that we are overlooking strategies employed by older women in Southern nations to live comfortably with the beginning phases of menopause. Rather than exploring the degree to which holistic traditional foods may buffer the so-called menopause syndrome, we place undue emphasis on medical interventions, such as estrogen replacement therapy. Instead of learning from traditional cultures about how women can positively experience these events, we have forsaken the cultural richness of human experiences in many Southern nations and are looking to the West for answers.

So profound are these dependency values that women themselves, having absorbed them, contribute to their promotion. In a culture constructed upon the complicity between the confluence of silence and submission, on the one hand, and philosophical misogyny, on the other, Chinese and other non-Western women not only are oppressed but also support their own oppression through the feelings of spiritual resignation that are dispersed throughout their societies (Chow, 1991). Western culture also contributes to the affirmation of womanhood only through the man's world. For example, a wife's adoption of her husband's name upon marriage is an alien custom that has been perpetuated by Western cultures in most traditional African societies (Mazrui, 1986). Traditionally, the women of Africa, my mother among them, retain their own names upon marriage. This is a legacy of the traditional African custom that helps to establish the individual within his or her own family lineage.

One aspect of the dimensions of health-seeking behavior that we have yet to explore concerns how the age gap between couples in Africa affects decision making in the household. In cultures that place emphasis on seniority and aging in decision making, a wife who is much younger than her husband does not necessarily have much decision-making power in the household. Such hierarchy of authority is usually a function of cultural values and reality, albeit to the disadvantage of women. The promotion of equity and independence in this context may not prove as practical as an exploration of strategies to bridge the spousal age gap while educating the family and community about women's need for autonomy. People, mostly men, have often reduced the problem of women to a problem of complementarity, with the excuse that the liberation of Black people in general is far more important than the liberation of women (Thiam, 1986). For example, the debate about abortion is nothing more than religious persecution of women. The same churches that are ready to demonize women for making choices are curiously quiet and have passively reified both de facto and de jure polygyny—a choice that privileges men. Here are two practices that go against the teachings of the church, both of which can potentially threaten the life of a woman, but only one places the woman as the ultimate decision maker, and many people, including some women, want to stop her. According to Minh-ha (1991), "Freedom written by a man is understood immediately as freedom; the same word coming from a woman must be clarified if she doesn't want freedom to be understood as licentiousness" (p. 122).

These are issues that must be considered on the macro level while we continue to deal with issues of individual and family health attitudes and behavior relative to health promotion and disease prevention. Throughout the nineteenth century, the British military in India was concerned only with maintaining an efficient and "healthy" army made up of men who had "natural" sexual desires that needed to be fulfilled (Amos & Parmar, 1984). In 1993, a similar policy was maintained by the U.S. military, as illustrated by the institutionalization of a regular supply of "healthy" Thai and Hawaiian female commercial sex workers for its men in uniform. Such commodification of women by governments is further evidence of postcolonial oppression.

## Sexuality and the Discourse on Womanhood

The masculinized construction of blame and sexual being has placed the responsibility of controlling the spread of sexually transmitted diseases (STDs) on women. Strategies designed to control STDs such as AIDS must take cognizance of the social contexts in which they are operating and must fully appreciate the weight of cultural tradition in structuring the social/sexual relationships between men and women. The folktales earlier related by Achebe are particularly applicable here. They capture the extent to which traditional cultures tend to function on similar terrain with other cultures at any given time, even though the cultures may be operating at different locations. For example, women have been (and still are, in some cultures) held responsible for the sexes of their babies. Therefore, women's humanity is affirmed not only by their ability to have children but by their ability to have male children.

A discussion of the issue of sexuality in the African context is incomplete without mention of the role of men in providing a collective solution. For an indigent African American woman, sex may serve as barter for the financial support of a male partner (Mays & Cochran, 1988). A woman may place more value on securing food and shelter for herself and her children than on practicing safer sex. Moreover, negotiating condom use with a sexual partner, for example, sometimes creates the perception of promiscuity. If a woman asks her male partner to use a condom, she is implying either that he has been "immoral" or that she is amoral. If she implies that she has been sexually permissive, she may risk rejection by her male partner; if she implies that he has been sexually permissive she risks his anger and outrage (Nichols, 1990). "In Nigeria, in each of the three major regional languages, Hausa, Igbo and Yoruba, corresponding to different ethnicities, the phrase used for STDs may be translated as 'women's diseases' " (Kisekka & Otesanya, 1990, quoted in Seidel, 1993, p. 180). HIV prevention efforts need to recognize that sexual activity occurs within a social context, and that only interventions that are presented within an interpersonal decision-making framework may prove effective (Cochran, 1990; Mays & Cochran, 1988).

The reasons many women do not use condoms or do not negotiate condom use are related to sex role socialization and social class issues. In the United States, although it might seem that the inability of women to use or negotiate the use of condoms contributes to the maintenance of the imbalance in the male-female relationship, this female powerlessness is better understood in the larger context of the economic security, the sex-ratio imbalance, and the meaning of sex experienced by African American women (Cochran, 1990; Fullilove, Fullilove, Haynes, & Gross, 1990; Nichols, 1990). As Seidel (1993) notes, "Life-saving strategies, negotiation and self-expression need to come through demystification and empowerment, and through economic and political leverage" (p. 181). This can be accomplished through government support for programs designed to address the disadvantaged position of women. If the PEN-3 model is used, positive, existential, and negative beliefs can be identified to ensure appropriate programmatic intervention. Examples of positive beliefs and actions in this context are cultural rituals in which women engage to prepare young girls for and to celebrate the passage into womanhood. An example of an existential practice is women's gender-related role as traders, which, if equitably rewarded socially, culturally, and economically, can prove to be positive. An example of negative beliefs and practices is the custom of discouraging young girls from becoming high achievers because of concern over their difficulty in finding husbands.

## Policy Implications

It appears that government policies target women only indirectly, through their children or their potential motherhood. A good example is the secondary focus on women found in child survival initiatives. Women are targeted in these programs to take responsibility for the improved health conditions of their children, not because women are considered worthy of such focus, but because their survival is inextricably tied to the survival of their children. Specific programs aimed at child survival, such as growth monitoring, oral rehydration therapy, breast-feeding/birth spacing, and immunization, rely for their success on the involvement of women. Although the focus on child survival is laudable, it would appear that a focus on family survival, particularly women's survival, is more crucial, because children are part of families, and the reality is that women are often the caretakers of their families.

Even when programs are designed to focus on the health concerns of women, they are still tied to the survival of children. An example is the Safe Motherhood Initiative, which, although admirable, particularly in light of the high rate of maternal mortality in African countries, often does not address the social and environmental conditions that shape women's status in a community and society. Factors such as women's degree of autonomy within the family structure, leverage for resource acquisition such as property rights, and decision-making role relative to sex role and reproductive rights all mediate women's health status long before, during, and long after pregnancy. Therefore, improving the health conditions of women within the context of patriarchal hegemony should be the focus of health policies, so that women's health can be addressed as women's health rather than only as mothers' health. The issue is not that there is too much emphasis on the health concerns of children, but that there is too little emphasis on the health concerns of women.

## Conclusion

The condition of women in a society can always be predicted by the overall status of women in that society. Therefore, programs aimed at improving women's health should commence with issues of equity for young girls. Low health status among women in a society not only affects the health of that society's children and youth but serves as an obstacle to the full participation of women in the development process. The absence of policies directed toward ameliorating the inequity in women's health will eventually lead to failed programs for children and youth. In Chapter 6, I address the health concerns of children and youth.

## Notes

1. Reprinted by permission of *Ms.* magazine, copyright © 1993.
2. Copyright © 1993 by The New York Times Company. Reprinted by permission.

# 6

# The Cultural Production of Healthy Children and Youth

Omonkaro—A child comes first.
Omonsigho—A child is more valuable than money.
Omonsefe—A child is more valuable than wealth.
Omonrotionmwan—A child is one's kin.
Omonragbon—A child is the world.

*common names in Edo (Benin, Nigeria)*

The naming of a child among the Edos of Nigeria, as well as many other groups in Africa, marks important cultural rituals within the family. Whether or not the naming of a child is marked by a ceremony, the selection of the name itself within the cultural context is never random. The name is designed to establish a specific historical trajectory as mediated by culture in the life of the family. The naming of children is symbolic of how different extended families try to reproduce themselves within their cultural codes and meaning. In this chapter, I define *youth* broadly as that period in an individual's life between childhood and adulthood. This period may include preteen, teen, and some postteen years. In many African cultures, individuals at these ages are often referred to as young adults, because there is no term equivalent to *adolescent* or *youth* in many languages. A teenaged person is usually referred to as *the young male child* or *the young female child.*

Children and youth foreground the constitution and meaning of the extended family in Africa. Therefore, an understanding of the role of children within African culture would be incomplete without an adequate contextualizing of the construction and functions of the extended family as a cultural production. Many reasons have been offered in the literature to explain why Africans have many children, principal among which are that children provide a cheap labor pool in agrarian societies and that high infant mortality rates lead to the naturalizing of multiparous desire. Explanatory models that problematize high birthrates and attempt to offer solutions often focus only on economic outcomes. Although it is important to consider individual income levels when addressing family size and structure, it is equally important to balance economics with psychosocial, cultural, and spiritual dimensions of family formation. Although high infant mortality rates are undeniable in many parts of Africa, the desire to have many children is equally evident among nonagrarians who live in a "First World" environment within "Third World" societies. Thus it is customarily understood that children form the core of what constitutes a family in most African contexts.

## The Context of Family

In Nigeria, for example, most "professionals" (e.g., university professors) have larger families than do their counterparts in Northern nations. It would appear that not even "enlightened" professionals are impervious to the cultural and psychosocial influences of their society. Surveys that constantly show the desire for fewer children among youths in secondary schools are quick to credit family planning programs for such reported expectations. Those who conduct the surveys, however, fail to recognize that similar expectations were expressed by many of today's parents who now have relatively large families. Expectations may be individually constructed on the basis of social formations as understood at a particular point in time, but reality is collectively produced on the basis of many factors that are not always within the individual's immediate control yet influence the individual, both consciously and subconsciously.

The survival of the child is very much dependent on the survival of the family, particularly of the mother. It is said in Africa that an orphan is any child without a mother. To the extent that African mothers are the primary caretakers of children, mothers' well-being is inextricably bound to the well-being of children. Attempts to address children's well-being have led to such international health projects as child survival programs instituted under the strong support of international donor agencies. Some international health experts question the rationale for such vertical programs (vertical in the sense that they tend to stand alone), because these programs tend to overlook the myriad factors affecting the health of children. Furthermore, the factors that influence the desired number of children, how the wife/mother in the family negotiates her decisions, and the role that family support has on the financial responsibilities assumed by the husband all affect the number of children planned and whether or not those children will survive and have economic, cultural, and social support.

## Health Issues and Services

The scarcity and unequal distribution of health facilities and services and limited economic and human resources have produced different levels and rates of infant and childhood diseases across the globe. Of every 100 children born in Africa, 12 die within their first year. In contrast, the infant mortality rate is 1-2 out of 100 in the United States (except for the African Americans and other minorities) and other Northern nations (U.N. Development Programme, 1993).

International health communities' efforts have been galvanized by increased understanding of the various benefits of child survival projects and the possibilities of removing various impediments that may thwart the potential achievements of these efforts. Two major child survival projects are the Extended Program on Immunization (EPI) and programs promoting oral rehydration therapy (ORT). EPI is an ambitious effort to establish universal immunization against six common childhood diseases—measles, tetanus, pertussis, polio, diphtheria, and tuberculosis. ORT programs utilize a three-tiered strategy to combat life-threatening diarrhea in infants: (a) administration of a simple solution of sugar and salts, (b) continued feeding through a diarrhea episode, and (c) referral, when appropriate. ORT replenishes the water and electrolytes lost from the body during a diarrhea episode through application of a simple, effective, low-cost solution. This child survival strategy also includes preventive disease techniques, such as hand washing, breast-feeding, and immunization. Thus ORT and EPI are complementary strategies.

However, regardless of the goodness of such projects' intent, the approach to the implementation of ORT programs and EPI epitomizes Western bias: Program administrators typically see only a problem to be solved and never acknowledge that the people involved may actually have their own method for overcoming it, given the right circumstances. Quite often, it is the circumstances that favor the disease's occurrence, progression, and recurrence that need to be checked. For example, David Werner (1989) has warned against undue reliance on ORT packets, because this only creates dependence. Instead of placing emphasis on teaching parents how to mix oral rehydration solution at home, using local implements and ingredients, most ORT programs encourage the use of prepared solution packets. New Western-based industries are now establishing rehydration solution manufacturing plants in African countries. One of the immediate negative consequences of these developments is the perception among many people that the ORT packets contain a cure for diarrhea rather than the premixed ingredients of a simple rehydration solution that can also be produced at home. This perception in turn has caused many to lose confidence in the value of ORT. To address these concerns, the PEN-3 model has been used as a guiding framework (the application of the model to child survival programs is discussed in Chapter 3).

Even when programs are successful in increasing the number of children who live beyond the age of 5, the years that follow are critical for these children's development, and this issue is often not addressed programmatically. In many societies, as youth enter adolescence they are seen mainly in terms of their problems rather than as active members of society. In Southern countries "street kids" are a current focus, as homeless children are in the West. Whereas proposed solutions in the West focus on engaging youth in activities that will keep them focused and free of boredom, in Africa the emphasis should be on creating jobs (Fanon, 1968).

## Cultural Construction of Youth

*Adolescent* is a term that is anchored in the medicalization of human growth and transformation. As this term is a signifier that foregrounds such negative characteristics as out-of-control behavior, irresponsibility, indecisiveness, and fatalism, it is not surprising that many programmatic efforts directed at adolescents are designed to address a "natural deficit" that is believed to be inevitably present in this group. Thus the word *adolescent* has several meanings—medical, cultural, political, legal, social, and historical. Whether adolescents are perceived negatively or positively, health promotion and disease prevention approaches directed toward them must be grounded in cultural realities.

In some societies, for example, a close relationship between a father and his son is believed to be optimal for the psychosocial well-being of the adolescent/youth. Such a relationship is commonly typified in the West by statements such as "My son is my best friend," and vice versa. Although close relationships between parents and children are also a goal in many African countries, such relationships translate to healthy and mutually enriching interactions and yet do not typify the notion of "friendship" as understood in the West. When I was growing up in Nigeria, the idea of (for instance) throwing a ball around with my father would have been as strange to me as it would have been to him. Yet I had the closest of relationships with my father at the same time I had good friends among my peers. The need to engage in leisure activities with one's child, such as playing ball, is a Western concept that has no social value within the cultural milieu in which I was nurtured. Within the African context, parents are expected to remain parents; children are expected to find their friends within their peer group. This culturally based family interaction pattern is particularly salient given the average number of children in African families and the centrality of children in these families. As we recognize the economic benefit of having fewer children, we should also recognize the sociopsychological and cultural benefits of having many children within this context. Such contextualization of family size is vital if we are to debate and make recommendations about "appropriate" family size.

It should be noted here that there are certain disadvantages to having few children, even in the West. Increasing numbers of individuals in cultures in which small family size is the norm are tending to engage in professionalization of extended family in the form of group therapy or support groups. Having no elders in one's family to advise one can also lead to professionalization of friendship in the form of counselors and/or therapists. The economic disadvantage (economic status being the core of Western notions of living) notwithstanding, there are notable social, psychological, and cultural benefits of having many children that we must not overlook in addressing the issue of family size in African cultural groups. The goal in deciding appropriate family size is to maintain a balance in all the important forces that shape the culture at a particular time.

The years that mark the bridge between childhood and adulthood are a very important evolutionary experience in individual growth and development. With so much negativity about the term *adolescent*, given its medicalized origin, perhaps a better term is *youth*. The youth of Africa today face more social and developmental challenges than do their parents. The often conflicting value systems of their culture and of Western culture have complicated their decision making and their ability to withstand environmental pressures to make healthy decisions. The confluence of the African top-down hierarchy of information flow and the top-down information flow within the school systems, which are borrowed from the West, has prestructured the youth to only receive information, never to produce it.

Youth may not be independent of family and societal institutions, such as schools, but they do function under the changing traditional values and customary practices of their environment. When tradition is wrongly viewed as a static state, with the necessary knowledge for its function stored in the minds of the elderly men and women in the society, the youth of Africa are often seen as divorced from traditional values and hence are assumed to be the products of modern values. Contemporary African youth do represent a confluence of traditional African culture and Western modern values, but although they are constantly exposed to Western values through the media, their interpretations of these values are often based on their interactions with, and their relationships with, their families, and family relationships are often characterized by experiences that are based in traditional culture. Furthermore, young people may not fully understand or acknowledge the degree to which certain of their behaviors manifest their cultural experiences. Thus the extent to which a young person acknowledges that his or her behaviors are grounded in traditional culture may be dependent on many factors, such as the opportunity for exposure to other cultural values, who the youth is communicating with and what the youth perceives that person to represent, and the culture of reference the youth believes that person represents.

## Health Behaviors

Social responsibility, which includes responding strictly to family dictates, is still a major expectation most parents have of their children. This responsibility is an important reason parents screen the friends their children choose. As regards sexuality and preventing sexually transmitted diseases, youths are more likely than adults to be influenced by referent group normative values. Peer pressure to engage in high-risk sexual and drug-related behaviors may be more prominent in inner-city neighborhoods in Western countries, thus increasing the difficulty of communicating about AIDS (Morales, 1987). In the United States, for example, the images of African American males have been exaggerated such that stereotypical notions of sexuality have been internalized by young African American men (Davis & Cross, 1979; Wyatt, Strayer, & Lobitz, 1976). Appearing to be concerned about contracting HIV or using condoms during sexual intercourse may be inconsistent with this cultural norm. In fact, sanctions may be directed at those who attempt to engage in health-promoting behaviors (Fisher, 1988). Reference group identification and its resulting social influence may, therefore, be a powerful force in shaping behavior among African American youth. Thus a peer-directed intervention may be useful in providing credible and positive role models and in creating a network of support to encourage the adoption and maintenance of self-protective behaviors.

However, youth are products of their environments, and they can be expected to behave in positive ways only as far as the support of adult guidance and their society makes possible. In this context, concern for sexuality decisions must be examined against such social mediators as unemployment and the relevance of the education and skills training youth receive to function in their society. Beyond these social concerns, there are social and cultural expectations that affect girl and boys differently. Young girls are faced with the pressure to experiment sexually just as boys are, but with the added burden of having to bear the brunt of the responsibility should unwanted pregnancy result. Unwanted pregnancy is perhaps the single most important event that can take place in a young woman's life; it is certain to limit and can sometimes completely derail her future prospects.

The pressure on young women to engage in sexual activity comes not only from young men but in many cases from older men who take advantage of the disadvantaged economic conditions of young women in their society to lure those women into sex. These men, often referred to as sugar daddies (*sour daddies* would be a more appropriate term), are responsible for significant numbers of teenage pregnancies in many African societies. The scenario is usually played out thus: A young woman is enticed with money to engage in sex with an older man and becomes pregnant; the man leaves, looking for other prey; the young woman withdraws from school or other activities that would have prepared her for a good future and has her baby. Such cases happen all over the world, although they may be more pronounced in many Southern nations. Any policy designed to address the problems of youth in Africa must seek to criminalize the role these "sugar daddies" play in truncating the life possibilities of the women they exploit.

Using the PEN-3 method, we can identify positive, existential, and negative beliefs and practices associated with the health of young people. One positive area is the degree of curiosity found in youth and their willingness to learn, provided they are exposed to positive stimuli. An example of an existential practice is youths' reliance on adult figures for direction. An example of a negative belief is the common attitude among young people that they are impervious to disease or injury.

## Conclusion

If, as the American Indian adage says, "we have not inherited the land from our ancestors, we are borrowing it from our children," then we owe our children a great debt. Children and youth represent our future possibilities. To the extent that we fail them, we have failed ourselves. With so much emphasis on child survival, we must remember that it is also critical that we prepare our youth to make the smooth transition to adulthood.

The social and cultural production of youth in Africa places youth within the context of family with certain responsibilities. Any discussion of the issue of youth is incomplete without special attention to the differential concerns of female youth and the role older men play in perpetuating their marginal status. This concern is one that transcends geographic and regional boundaries.

# 7

# Contextualizing the Health Praxis of African Americans

> Unable to call upon the power of ancestors, because one does not know them; without an ideology of heritage, because one does not respect one's own prophets; the person is like an ant trying to move a large piece of garbage only to find that it will not move.
>
> *Molefi K. Asante,* Afrocentricity, *1987*

> You have to position yourself somewhere in order to say something at all. Thus, we cannot do without that sense of our own positioning that is connoted by the term ethnicity. And the relation that peoples of the world now have to their own past is, of course, part of the discovery of their own ethnicity. They need to honor the hidden histories from which they've been not taught to speak. They need to understand and revalue the traditions and inheritances of cultural expression and creativity. And in that sense, the past is not only

---

AUTHOR'S NOTE: This chapter contains portions of three previous publications: my chapter "Health Promotion and Disease Prevention Strategies for African Americans," in R. L. Braithwaite and S. E. Taylor (Eds.), *Health Issues in the Black Community,* copyright © 1992 by Jossey-Bass; my article, coauthored with Ralph DiClemente, Gina Wingood, and Agatha Lowe, "HIV / AIDS Education and Prevention Among African-Americans: A Focus on Culture," *AIDS Education and Prevention,* 4, 267-276, copyright © 1992 by Guilford Press; and my chapter, coauthored with Agatha Lowe, "Improving the Health Status of African-Americans: Empowerment as Health Education Intervention," in I. L. Livingston (Ed.), *Handbook of Black American Health: The Mosaic of Conditions, Issues, Policies and Prospects,* copyright © 1994 by Greenwood Press, an imprint of Greenwood Publishing Group. All are used by permission.

> a position from which to speak, but it is also an absolutely necessary resource in what one has to say.
>
> *Stuart Hall, "Ethnicity: Identity and Difference," 1991*

Some professionals have suggested that there is no authentic African American culture, and therefore alternative theories and perspectives on the health-seeking behaviors of African Americans are unnecessary. Some of those who do believe in the existence of an African American culture apparently view it as only a deviant variation of the majority culture (Aldous, 1969; Parker & Kleiner, 1969). Further, there are some who believe that even though there are some differences between African American culture and the dominant White culture, there is no value or benefit to be found in accentuating the differences without according equal coverage to other groups (West, 1993)—that is, confronting the issue of multiculturalism. However, there is strong evidence that African Americans stand to benefit more from health promotion and disease prevention programs when those programs are conducted in ways that affirm and legitimate African Americans' cultural codes and meanings. Such affirmation of differences in health promotion activities in African American communities should be promoted (Airhihenbuwa & Pineiro, 1988).

The project of legitimating and affirming the voices of African Americans' cultural space has been a focus of research and practice by scholars of African American culture. One example of this cultural project is Afrocentric theory, which is anchored in a belief in the centrality of Africanity in any analysis involving African culture and behavior. For instance, as Asante (1987) notes, "The communicationist who defines a speech as an uninterrupted spoken discourse demonstrates either a disregard or ignorance of the African tradition of speech, much as Leslie Fiedler showed a purely European conception of fiction when he contended that romance was a central theme in literature" (p. 6). According to James Stewart (1992), Afrocentric theory tends to fall into two basic categories. The first is the

> 'strong claim'—the assertion that the liberation of peoples of African descent requires a psychological reorientation that focuses on reconstructing selected aspects of traditional African psychology, values and behaviors in the present. The second is the 'weak claim'—the position that liberation requires that top priority be assigned to the interests of peoples of African descent in social and political intercourse with other collectives. (p. 35)

African American cultural scholars have consistently challenged the application of traditional models based on White culture for recommending treatment and/or behavior change targeted at health promotion and disease prevention among African Americans. Research evidence confirms the lack of congruence of these practices with the African American experience, lifestyle, and culture (Jackson, 1983b; Leonard & Jones, 1980). In response to these deficits, some researchers have proposed African- and African American-based personality and treatment models (Baldwin, 1981; Nobles, 1980; Parham & Helms, 1985). Consequently, new approaches for educational and behavioral change models have been advanced.

Afrocentric scholars tend to agree that African American values are a confluence of African heritage and the American experience (Jackson, 1983a; Nobles, 1980). Although the focus for many years has been on the American experience (Jackson, 1983a), scholars such as Asante (1983, 1987) emphasize retained African values and behavioral patterns. Examples include the extended family, the belief that all the aunts and uncles are responsible parents of all their nieces and nephews, the belief in collectivism as opposed to individualism, and respect for age (Allen, 1978). A lifestyle of acquiescence to nature rather than challenging it and an emphasis on oral tradition are also hallmarks of African values.

Jackson (1983b) notes: "Cultural theories in Black psychology are characterized generally by an emphasis on 'wellness' or normality instead of psychopathology. The focus on normality in turn is based on an African value system" (p. 20). Theoretical formulations are relevant only to the extent that cultural values are recognized and incorporated (E. T. Hall, 1977). Because health behaviors are culture bound, primary prevention efforts that address preventable disease and illness must emerge from a knowledge and understanding of the target culture so that health interventions are culturally sensitive and linguistically appropriate (Braithwaite & Lythcott, 1989).

Stewart (1989) has called for the development and prioritizing of a grand theory of Africology based on a full understanding of the nature of history, time, space, and technology in Afrocentric terms. He argues that our political and intellectual efforts should be devoted to restructuring community ties and translating the language of African American intellectual elites into the language of African American popular culture. Such a framework will capture the beliefs of Africans and African Americans in postmodern history (Asante, 1987). However, some scholars, such as Marable (1993), have questioned the wisdom of analyzing African American culture and behavior based solely on African culture: "African, in effect, represents only one-half of the dialectical consciousness of African American people. Blacks are also legitimately Americans and, by our suffering, struggle and culture, we have a destiny within this geographical and political space equal to or stronger than that of any white American" (p. 121). In the words of Angela Davis (1992), "There is no simple or unitary way to look at expressions of Black nationalism or essentialism in contemporary cultural forms" (p. 320).

It is not my intent here to debate what constitutes the production of African American culture in the mid-1990s, but it is worth noting that even after African Americans' many years of lived experience in the United States, there still remain many compelling similarities between African Americans and Africans with regard to certain cultural codes and meanings in actions and behaviors. Such behaviors can be found in choices and values assigned to foods, the importance of orature and oracy in communication, and the use of traditional healing, all of which are important in the development of health promotion and disease prevention programs. In this context, this chapter focuses on the degree to which African Americans' health conditions can benefit from culturally appropriate paradigms that are grounded in historical correctness rather than mere political correctness.

In spite of efforts to understand cultural values as they relate to personal behaviors, little attention has been given to the development of a culturally appropriate paradigm for health promotion in the African American community. Currently, culturally sensitive educational and behavioral change models for health promotion in African

American communities tend to be based primarily on the Caucasian experience. Attempts to make these programs culturally appropriate tend to rely on the individual and family psychology of African Americans. A major shortcoming of these models is the failure to ground personal crises in the social political context within which the individual has to function. It is critical to establish a balance between behavior the individual is capable of changing and the social-political factors in the environment that must be managed before those changes are meaningful and sustainable. The outcome is that these approaches offer no models for translating known cultural and psychological realities into a working framework that could guide the development of culturally appropriate health promotion and disease prevention programs in African American communities. Myers and King (1983) present a dialectic crisis-conflict model for understanding mental health outcomes in the development of the African American child. The uniqueness of this model is manifested in its recognition not only of the significance and depth of the personal crisis faced by the African American child but of the etiological significance of the undeveloped consciousness in the victim of the fundamental social contradictions that he or she faces.

Given the faulty premise that African American culture is not different from White culture, it has been easy for Eurocentrists, health professionals and laypeople alike, to delude themselves into thinking that they are familiar with African American culture in all of its aspects (Jackson, 1983a). The consequences of such a mind-set include failed health care programs for African American communities—programs that may have been conceived out of genuine concern for the communities, but that have been methodologically and theoretically flawed. There is no doubt that the failure to recognize the cultural inadequacies of traditional models, so as to promote and educate people to use alternative models, has contributed significantly to the profound disparity in health status between African Americans and the White population. "The degree to which African Americans perceive the 'odds against them' as manageable or overwhelming will depend to a significant degree on the transactional competency and success of their parents, the competence of the role models in their primary community of competency, and, finally, on the availability and accessibility of resources and supports to help them in their coping efforts" (Myers & King, 1983, p. 294).

Although socioeconomic status influences health outcomes, racial and cultural differences are also associated with the low health status of African Americans (Airhihenbuwa, 1989a). In the words of Derrick Bell (1992), "What we now call the 'inner city' is, in fact, the American equivalent of South African homelands. Poverty is less the source than the status of men and women who, despised because of their race, seek refuge in self-rejection" (p. 4). Low economic status is linked with poor health status, and other factors, such as structural discrimination and institutional racism, favor the disproportionate representation of African Americans in low-income groups, which ultimately results in their poor health status. A focus on individual income fails to address the social context and environment in which a disproportionate number of African Americans find themselves (Auslander, Haire-Joshu, Houston, & Fisher, 1992). Even among African Americans whose income levels are the same as those of the majority White population, many other factors—such as total assets, housing, prior socioeconomic status, and social mobility—influence health status (Kumanyika & Golden, 1991).

A position paper adopted by the American Public Health Association's Governing Council in 1974 refers to racism as an established characteristic of the health care delivery system (cited in Muller, 1985). The impact of health service accessibility problems on African American families is a reflection of the poor quality of care they receive. When choices for available services are limited or nonexistent, the quality of services is hardly ever questioned by public policy makers. The goal of the public health system in the United States should be the achievement of social equity in the health status of all Americans. The discussion that follows examines some of the reasons gaps persist between the races in the delivery of health services.

## Disparities in Health Status

Disparities in health status between African Americans and Whites have long been and continue to be realities in the United States. Blacks of both sexes and in all age groups are more likely than Whites to be ill or to die prematurely. The 1989 mortality data for Black men showed a continued reduction in life expectancy and no change for both sexes, in sharp contrast to the extension of life by 0.4 years for Whites of both sexes ("Health Trends," 1992). Age-specific excess deaths for Blacks compared with Whites in 1991 ranged from 64% for persons aged 15-25 to 11% for persons 65 years and older (Fingerhut & Makuc, 1992).

A Black baby is more than twice as likely as a White infant to die before his or her first birthday (Edelman, 1989). In 1989, the infant mortality rate for Whites was 8.2 per 1,000 live births, compared with 17.7 per 1,000 for Blacks ("Health Trends," 1992). The gap is even wider (8.1 for Whites and 18.6 for Blacks) when the mother's race is used to classify infant mortality rate. The proportion of low-birth-weight infants among Black mothers is almost three times that of Whites. The 1989 rate of 13.3% (compared with 5.7% for Whites) has been increasing yearly from 12.7% in 1980 (U.S. Department of Health and Human Services, 1991).

Effective use of available, accessible, and affordable preventive services can significantly improve maternal and child health. A major factor responsible for the disparity in health conditions of African Americans compared with Whites is the underrepresentation of African Americans as health providers. Proctor and Rosen (1981) found that African Americans may not always express racial preferences or expectations regarding their health care providers, but when they do, they indicate a desire to be seen by African American health care providers. Bonding along racial lines, even for an impersonal health care provider, suggests the strength of the historical experience of a group. To the extent that physicians rely on a patient's "will to live" as critical to the patient's prognosis, particularly after complicated surgery, the patient's "will to perceive" an acceptable health care provider is equally critical. Thus we must take seriously the patient's assumptions about the competence of such a person on the basis of his or her racial identity and its compatibility with that of the patient. Even if an African American patient is not seen by an African American physician in a medical facility, the patient's knowledge of the presence of an African American practitioner in that facility can help to alleviate some apprehensions he or she may have about services. People who share similar cultural patterns, values, experiences, and problems are more likely to feel comfortable with and to understand each other (Levy, 1985).

Whitehead (1992) and others have proposed a cultural model (the cultural systems paradigm) designed to centralize culture in the understanding of the decisions and behaviors of African American individuals and families. This model has been useful for the conceptualization of a holistic approach to understanding culturally based food choices by African Americans. This model also takes into account the social political and environmental context within which individuals function.

The need to examine the personal or cultural health beliefs of African Americans is increasingly critical. For example, teenage pregnancy is an issue that has received increasing public attention in the past decade. In the development of health interventions targeting teen pregnancies, the assumption is usually made that all such pregnancies are unwanted. Consequently, interventions tend to concentrate on recommendations of birth control methods for all teenagers. Such recommendations, however, are totally irrelevant for teenagers whose pregnancies are planned, an increasing number of whom are African American. Programs aimed at preventing pregnancies among teenagers who want to become pregnant need to examine and deal with societal failures that condition these children to want to have children. Children having children is one concern, but children *wanting* to have children is another—there is no worse evidence that a society has failed its youth.

Dealing head-on with the truth of this individual construction of reality is not to suggest an endorsement of such reality, but to focus on the manifestations of human growth and transformation. In other words, accepting the truth of wanted pregnancies among teenagers can allow interventionists to explore why these teenagers want to have children. Both wanted and unwanted teenage pregnancies have important policy implications. Health and social practices are usually manifestations of several forces that collectively shape individuals' cultural beliefs and individual life experiences. In the case of children wanting to have and having children, the interventions that may be most successful in the long run may be those that concentrate on the factors—such as failed government policies, high rates of unemployment, and various forms of marginalization and discrimination—that have contributed to teenagers' feeling that they have no other future.

## Problems in Health Institutions

The notion of health care as a delivery system is a myth that continues to be perpetuated. The health care industry does not deliver health care, at least not to the African American community. The rendering of health care services (to those who can afford them) should be demystified and presented for what it is—a medical production. Once we understand that the health care system is a medical production, we can place it in relation to its political economy, that is, who produces it and how the producers control the costs of the services they render, who consumes them and how that consumption is rationed, and who has little access to services and why this is the case. Recent U.S. health care reform proposals have emphasized structural access as critical to ensuring universal coverage. Although this seems reasonable, it does not address issues of corporate/societal responsibility by way of, for example, criminalization of billboard advertising for alcohol and tobacco products that targets minority communities, enhancement of historically Black medical schools' ability to increase the supply of African American health providers, and promotion of cultural sensitivity among health providers and health programs that are central to providing meaningful universal health coverage to African Americans and other non-White populations. Concerns about access must not be restricted only to dollar costs for coverage of care; equally important are the opportunity, emotional, and spiritual costs of unacceptable services.

These latter costs are evident in research findings concerning the indices of availability, acceptability, and affordability, as well as accessibility, of health care services for African Americans. An examination of the availability of health care resources reveals that the condition has worsened for African Americans since the U.S. Department of Health and Human Services published its 1985 task force report on the status of Black and minority health (cited in Hale, 1992). Indeed, in a 1988 response to that report issued by the Commission on Minority Participation in Education and American Life, the investigators concluded that the United States is "moving backward" in its efforts to secure equity for minority citizens (Jacob, 1989). Reductions in federal financing programs slowed the decentralization of health care resources through block grants and attenuated the increasing accessibility of health care services for minorities and the disadvantaged. For example, the Health Education-Risk Reduction Grants Program was cut by 25% as a consequence of the 1980s block grant policy (Kreuter, 1992).

Even when services are available, they may not be as accessible to Blacks as to Whites, because Black families are often faced with different barriers that complicate their access to health services. For instance, some physicians refuse to treat patients who are indigent (Davidson, 1982) and some refuse patients who are Black (Charatz-Litt, 1992). Other barriers include limited access to medical facilities, long waiting times at medical facilities, inconvenient medical office hours, and absence of privacy within public and private clinics and emergency rooms (Davidson, 1982).

The underrepresentation of Black professionals in the health care delivery system has complicated the problem of accessibility (Airhihenbuwa, 1989a). As of 1989, Blacks constituted 12.1% of the U.S. population, and 13.6% of the population aged 20 to 29, yet African Americans received only 5.3% of the medical degrees awarded in that year (Petersdorf, Turner, Nickens, & Ready, 1990). African Americans accounted for only 5.8% of the total number of doctorates awarded in health education between 1980 and 1988 (Airhihenbuwa et al., 1989). Of the total number of graduates from schools of public health in the 1981-1982 academic year, only 2.5% were Blacks (Airhihenbuwa et al., 1989). As noted above, Proctor and Rosen (1981) found that when Blacks have a preference, they express a desire to be attended to by Black health care providers. African American counseling clients in Miles and McDavis's (1982) research expressed finding comfort in the knowledge that there were Black counselors on the counseling staff. An increase in the number of Black health professionals might well improve accessibility and subsequently quality of health care delivery to Black clients. The presence of Black faculty in health education and other public health academic departments may directly or indirectly enhance the recruitment and, more important, the retention of Blacks in these programs (Airhihenbuwa et al., 1989).

Although increasing Black representation in the health care professions is important, of equal importance is an emphasis on cultural sensitivity among health care professionals. Medical schools and schools of public health need to offer courses that will prepare future health professionals to understand the differing cultural values and meanings of medical practice for their patients. Such education could be instrumental in breaking down the cycle of institutional racism. Structural discrimination and institutional racism are synergistically responsible, in large part, for the persistent disparity between Blacks and Whites in availability and accessibility of health services. This is evident in the ways the policies and practices of the White medical community negatively affect the health of African Americans (Charatz-Litt, 1992) as well as in the history of racism as an established characteristic of the health care system (Muller, 1985).

Discriminatory practices in health care availability and accessibility are often exacerbated by the limited resources of many African Americans. Investigators have documented the disproportionate decrease in income levels among Blacks compared with Whites. On the basis of constant dollars, 30% more Blacks than Whites had an annual income of less than $5,000 in 1987 than had occurred in 1970 (Horton & Smith, 1990). Today, 34% of African Americans are below the poverty level, compared with 11% of Whites (Auslander et al., 1992). Opportunity costs, or the synergy of time and money required to access available health services, are also a major barrier to health care for the economically disadvantaged (Airhihenbuwa, 1992).

Services that are available, accessible, and affordable must also be acceptable to patients. Racism has separated Blacks and Whites to the extent that many White health care professionals are unaware of the Black experience (of suffering and discrimination particularly) and the effect it has on Black people. This ignorance may prevent professionals from understanding both the cultural appropriateness of African American clients' behavior and the adaptive qualities of such behavior. White professionals may therefore discount the value of, or incorrectly label, the behavior of a Black client as abnormal. Conversely, ignorance of Black lifestyles may contribute to health care workers' tendency to attribute certain behaviors to racial differences when such behavior should be ascribed to personal malfunctioning and psychopathology.

Of the 10 leading causes of death in 1976, 50% were related to unhealthy behaviors or lifestyles, 20% to environmental factors, 20% to human ecological factors, and only 10% to inadequacies in health care (U.S. Surgeon General, 1979). Thus doctors have little or no control over many of the factors that make us ill or keep us well. By focusing on lifestyles, social conditions, and the physical environment, health educators have been successful at improving the health of the population (Airhihenbuwa, 1989a). Because the majority of Black clients receive care from White professionals, cultural differences often arise in doctor-patient relations. Many African Americans are suspicious of White health care institutions, at least in part because Blacks have historically been exploited for medical experimentation and demonstration (Jones, 1982; Pernick, 1985; Savitt, 1982).

Recent studies on health promotion and disease prevention have shown that improving self-esteem, building skills, and providing support are the three most important ways to promote positive health behavior change (Keeling, 1992). However, the improvement of self-esteem, building of skills, and provision of social support are all influenced by the degree to which individuals can influence other forces within their environments. The empowerment of individuals, groups, and communities rests upon their ability to understand and manage or at least function adequately within existing environmental forces. The next section explores strategies for promoting such abilities within the context of the African American family and community.

## Health Promotion/Education Interventions

Existing health promotion strategies for U.S. ethnic minority populations tend to be based on theories and frameworks drawn from the White population. Although these theories provide insights into human behavior in general, they are inadequate for the planning, implementation, and evaluation of health promotion and disease prevention programs for African American communities.

Health promotion and disease prevention programs that target individual behavior change must not absolve the government of its responsibility to provide a secure environment in which individuals have the opportunities and resources they need to make decisions and engage in positive activities that lead to improved self-esteem. Bandura (1977) has demonstrated that individuals' personal expectations of their ability to influence events in life (self-efficacy) determine whether they will initiate behavior to deal with particular situations, how much effort they will expend, and how long they will sustain the effort in the face of obstacles and aversive experiences. Those who believe they have the skills to cope will be more likely to use those skills if they have the resources to utilize them and the support and protection necessary to do so. Thus skill development among African Americans is pivotal to their empowerment within the context of having necessary supports and rewards from society.

Techniques used to facilitate the transition from powerlessness to empowerment among health care clients have embraced consciousness-raising, training in social competence that includes encouraging and accepting the client's definition of the problem, identifying and building upon existing strengths, analyzing how powerlessness is affecting the situation, identifying and using sources of power in the client's situation, the teaching of specific skills, mobilization of resources, and looking out for the client's welfare (Gutierrez, 1990). Another technique that should be developed is that of encouraging individuals and groups to work collectively toward changing negative policies and forces in their environments. The ideal modality for promoting empowerment is the small group, because it facilitates the use of such techniques as consciousness-raising, engaging in mutual aid, development of knowledge and skills, the modeling of behaviors, and problem solving. Individuals in small groups can evaluate their effectiveness in influencing others and can receive support as they learn and practice new skills. Their interpersonal skills can influence their ability to influence others, to work toward changing institutions and social structures, and to attain personal and collective goals (Gutierrez, 1990; Ozer & Bandura, 1990; Saegert, 1989). This is true whether the goal is empowering individuals or institutions. Groups also provide support through the change process, a format for obtaining concrete assistance, and a potential power base for future action (Gutierrez, 1990). The outcomes of empowerment include changes at individual, interpersonal, institutional, community, and societal levels.

African Americans in different parts of the United States are assuming responsibility for finding solutions to the health and social problems that affect them and their families, in spite of the structural and psychological barriers that consign a disproportionate number of them to the lowest socioeconomic strata of society. The greatest contribution the government can make is to remove the barriers that frustrate the efforts of grassroots organizations to facilitate the empowerment of the African American family, because the latter remains one of the strongest institutions in Black communities. The African American family must become a collaborator before programs can effectively meet the needs of the Black population (Airhihenbuwa, 1989a).

Collectively and independently, African American family members must develop the skills necessary to lead to positive health behavior change. Health educators should help families to develop the skills they need for self-efficacy and empowerment. They can accomplish this by working with others in public health, particularly individuals of African descent (students as well as professionals), to identify and help address the needs of the community, as prioritized by the community. An example concerning food choices and food-related beliefs among African Americans, using the PEN-3 model, serves as an illustration. The application of the PEN-3 model allows health professionals to appreciate the social/environmental forces that may promote or threaten the success of positive health actions. Some positive health beliefs and actions among African Americans concerning food include the customs of eating green vegetables and eating at home with one's family. Existential health beliefs and actions include the drinking of pot liquor (the juice from cooked vegetables) and the belief that eating is a spiritual experience. Examples of negative beliefs and actions include the eating of greasy foods and the attitude that one has no control over what is cooked at home.

While addressing individual behaviors, interventionists should also recognize environmental forces that may thwart individual efforts. An example of this is the availability of fast-food restaurants in most African American neighborhoods. This reality, coupled with the negative reinforcement of cigarette billboard advertising and liquor stores on every corner, represents forces that may require government intervention to control.

Preventive health initiatives can be introduced simultaneously with actions taken to address a community's prioritized needs, or after those needs have been addressed. The Black Students Leadership Network, for example, combines community service with political activism. This organization has worked to empower Blacks in housing projects to have control over the forces and decisions in their environment (e.g., influencing town council and community agencies' decisions about services provided in the community) that influence the destiny of their families and communities (Collison, 1992).

Sullivan (1989), a former U.S. secretary of health and human services, points out that one way to address the disproportionately high rates of infant deaths and deaths from chronic degenerative conditions among African Americans is through increased emphasis on health education and preventive care. This call for preventive strategies is appropriate and timely, but we must be cautious not to develop health promotion and disease prevention programs under the assumption that individuals have total control over the factors that influence their health. There is a tendency to believe that, given the right information, and perhaps the right circumstances, individuals will be willing and able to change their health conditions. Indeed, largely as a result of health promotion programs, many Americans now engage in a variety of risk-reduction activities and, as a result, some have experienced improvement in, for example, lipid profiles, protection against hypertension, and decrease in obesity, as well as healthier cardiovascular systems (Sprafka, Burke, Folsom, & Hahn, 1989). However, placing so much of the responsibility for health promotion and disease prevention on the individual has serious limitations (Becker, 1986; Lamarine, 1989). As Becker (1986) observes, the focus on the individual "enables us to ignore the more difficult, but at least equally important problem of the social environment, which both creates some lifestyles and inhibits the initiation of others" (p. 19).

The assumption that the distribution of information will result in changes in behavior is based on an assumption that the information is "correct" and/or unanimously acceptable. Yet the content of some health promotion messages can be misleading, or so confusing that individuals have difficulty sorting out the facts (e.g., the mixed messages we have received about caffeine in recent years). As Lamarine (1989) notes, the scientific bases of many recommended programs are not clearly established, and there is thus much misinformation distributed. For health education programs designed for African American communities the situation is even worse, particularly because cultural influences on health behavior (such as in food selection practices) are often ignored.

Individuals gain the ability to manipulate their environments by acquiring the skills to review information critically and by raising their levels of consciousness through the support of and sharing with friends and families. They are then better able to make appropriate decisions regarding health-enhancing activities. The decision-making task is a serious challenge, because avoiding most preventable diseases requires individuals to make lifelong changes, and failure to make those changes rarely results in immediate illness. Consequently, individuals whose daily survival is a struggle may perceive limited benefit in adopting lifelong patterns that involve abstention, for example, from eating certain foods, engaging in unprotected sexual intercourse, smoking, or alcohol use. It is for the benefit of accentuating the connection between an individual's livelihood and positive health practices that African Americans must be empowered to develop the skills and support they need to make positive health decisions. For African Americans, support, either within community groups or in the larger society, is essential to the promotion of changes at individual and group levels.

Overall, individual and group empowerment of African Americans benefits all of society, because African Americans who are empowered will have a greater sense of political efficacy, a greater desire for control over their environment, greater civic-mindedness, and a general belief that success results from internal rather than external factors. These outcomes, in time, will result in positive contributions to the improved health status of African Americans. Even when people of color tend to be race effacing in their cultural identities, their allegiance to their hitherto denied cultural heritages tends to become stronger in times of personal conflict and professional problems.

## Cultural Factors in Promoting Health

Culture represents a set or sets of shared behaviors and ideas that are symbolic, systematic, cumulative, and transmitted from generation to generation (Nobles, 1985). Culture comprises a vast structure of language, customs, knowledge, ideas, and values that provides people with a general design for living and patterns for interpreting reality. As a way to clarify the dynamics of ethnic minority cultures, I offer the metaphor of the U.S. educational and health care systems as a salad bowl, rather than as the melting pot it has long been imagined to be (Airhihenbuwa & Pineiro, 1988). The melting pot concept assumes that every culture in the United States is assimilated into the mainstream White Anglo-Saxon Protestant culture, forsaking previous cultural identity and heritage in the pursuit of sameness. It is this melting pot mentality that leads health professionals to disregard cultural differences as critical factors that must be considered in the development of health interventions. Consequently, they employ what they believe to be culturally universal solutions.

The salad bowl concept recognizes cultural diversity and the separate and unequal statuses of different groups in U.S. society. If a nation's people all share common customs, origin, history, and language, then the United States could be considered a country of many nations, including African Americans, Hispanic Americans, Asian Americans, and Native Americans. The salad bowl concept approaches heterogeneity with positive rather than negative connotations. Cultural differences affect health status and outcomes; therefore, health programs must be developed to address such differences. Acceptance of the salad bowl concept is significant for health education because it is necessarily prerequisite to the encouragement and development of culturally appropriate health programs.

## HIV/AIDS Prevention Among African Americans

The prevention of HIV infection among African American women presents particular problems for health educators. Behavior change strategies emphasize the use of condoms and spermicide, careful selection of partners, and abstention from sex. Programs attempt to provide women with the skills they need to negotiate with men for safer sex practices. Hankins (1990) argues that strategies based on empowering women to be more assertive in sexual negotiations are in themselves inadequate, because in both Northern and Southern countries, women "who are at higher risk for HIV acquisition do not have the power within sexual relationships to negotiate a change in the rules" (p. 444). Black women in particular run the risk of being abused (Mays & Cochran, 1988) or of being rejected by men if they try to put these strategies into practice. For some women, the risk of losing a partner may outweigh that of contracting HIV.

The control of pediatric AIDS among African Americans is difficult also. Childbearing in this culture is important to a woman's self-esteem; an HIV-positive woman may thus want to take the 30-60% chance that her child might not be infected. Further, such a woman may not be able to obtain an abortion even if she wants one, because of her HIV status (Mitchell, 1988). The societal powerlessness of African American women, coupled with poverty, discrimination, apparent lack of official interest in the presence of HIV infection in women, exclusion of women from some treatment programs for drug abuse and for AIDS, and lack of adequate maternity and other health services for women, has led to a rather pessimistic view about the possibility of changing the risks of infection for these women (N. K. Bell, 1989; Hankins, 1990).

Doyle, Smith, and Hosokawa (1989) used individual counseling, group educational sessions, and various media (radio, newsletters, churches, and community social gatherings) to transmit a variety of health messages to African Americans. They found "churches to be the most effective means of reaching the target group" (p. 62). Direct face-to-face contact was also effective, particularly when the person making the contact was culturally and socioeconomically similar to the targeted individual. Lau, Quadrel, and Hartman (1990) have shown that parental influence on the health behavior of young adult children is greater than that of the children's peers. The use of contraceptives by African American girls has been found to be more strongly influenced by the involvement of their mothers than by that of the girls' peers (Nathanson & Becker, 1986).

The African American family's influence on children's health and the strengths of African American women should form the basis for health education programs for African American families. The PEN-3 model can be used as the framework for planning health interventions in African American communities. Program planners must identify positive, existential, and negative socioeconomic, health, cultural, and environmental factors affecting Black families and shaping the development and maintenance of their health-seeking behaviors. Barriers to behavior change must also be a part of this analysis. Community members (both women and men) and agencies must be involved in planning, implementing, and evaluating programs targeted to that community. To be effective, messages must be persuasive; care must be taken that they not produce avoidance because of the fears they engender or because of their incompatibility with community group norms. Messages should address behaviors that individuals can change, and financial and other supports should be provided so that such change is possible.

Programs should be delivered by people who are credible to the community. This means that more African Americans must be recruited to become involved. Health messages must reach the people wherever they normally congregate: workplaces, homes, hair salons and barbershops, churches, bars, and streets. A concerted effort must be made to change the socioeconomic and other discriminatory health delivery practices affecting the African American family.

## Conclusion and Recommendations

Health promotion programs have been effective in helping individuals to decrease their risks of some diseases, such as cancer, cardiovascular problems, and hypertension. However, targeting individuals for most health promotion and disease reduction efforts without considering the effects of their environments may be counterproductive, because few have control over most environmental factors that influence them. Interventionists must manipulate the sociopolitical and environmental forces that influence health behavior within the context of the culture, utilizing source experts who can also serve as positive role models to influence behavior change (Airhihenbuwa, DiClemente, Wingood, & Lowe, 1992). Finally, to promote health-enhancing activities, all health professionals need to become advocates of the people for whom options are rapidly decreasing. For example, the fact that doctors are available in greater numbers where certain diseases have become rare has little to do with the doctors' ability to control or eliminate disease. It simply means that doctors deploy themselves as they like, more so than other professionals, and that they tend to gather where the climate is healthy, where the water is clean, and where people are employed and can pay for their services (Illich, 1976, p. 21). Health professionals need to focus on environmental and social factors that rob people of hope and dignity and that contribute to poverty and crime. If left unaddressed, these can become further contributors to the health risks of African Americans.

# 8

# Approaches to Health Promotion Beyond the Turn of the Century

> To know who you are is the beginning of wisdom. By achievements, Africans are the people of the day before yesterday. In potential, we are the people of the day after tomorrow. In between, we have been a pawn in other people's desire.
>
> *Ali A. Mazrui,* The Africans: A Triple Heritage, *1986*

Cultural imperialism is manifested in school curricula that hold up Western and European experiences as the only experiences of importance. Even when other histories, languages, and cultures are taught, the images and the instruments of learning are often designed such that they are rooted in the past; it seems that the achievements of other cultures are to be glorified only for their nostalgia value—they hold no future possibilities. There is often no attempt to connect any information about non-Western cultures with current political realities, power, and education. Persons who are the products of colonial/postcolonial realities are conditioned to believe that everything good about themselves and their cultures existed only in the past and should remain there (see Said, in Mariani & Crary, 1990). This has

AUTHOR'S NOTE: This chapter contains a brief portion of my article "Health Promotion and the Discourse on Culture: Implications for Empowerment," *Health Education Quarterly, 21*(3), 345-353. Copyright © 1994 by John Wiley & Sons, Inc., Publishers.

long been true for people of African descent all over the world, particularly in matters relating to health beliefs and practices.

The success of health promotion programs in Africa rests with the degree to which they are based on the sociocultural realities of Africans. "Economic and political control of a people can never be complete without cultural control, and here literal scholarly practice, irrespective of any individual interpretation and handling of the practice, fitted well the aim and the logic of the system as a whole" (Thiong'O, 1986, p. 93).

In a 1991 multiagency report on the future direction of health education, the International Union of Health Promotion and Education, the World Health Organization, and the U.S. Centers for Disease Control did not center on cultural issues as a critical element in the promotion of health. Some still believe that these issues ought simply to be acknowledged, not situated at the core of health promotion programs. At best, the agencies' report alludes to culture as one of several secondary factors to be considered in health promotion. This document fails to accent how culture informs the various domains and dimensions (personal, institutional, and societal) of health promotion. The absence of cultural appropriateness as a major theme in this important health education document is a terrible and unfortunate omission. To treat culture as a commonsense issue is to reinscribe the notion of universal truth in health, education, and development projects. Common sense is not common; it is relative and shaped by cultural landscapes and locations.

Food, water, and air, in correlation with the level of sociopolitical equality and the cultural mechanisms that make it possible to keep a population stable, play decisive roles in determining how healthy adults feel and at what ages they tend to die (Illich, 1976, p. 20).

## Health Education and Empowerment

Cultural empowerment in health promotion and education can be an effective tool that enriches the production and acquisition of knowledge for interventionists and their audiences. The emphasis on participation of people in group action and dialogue is critical to the extent that interventionists do not assume the population is powerless at both the micro and the macro levels of decision making. The process must not assume that the community lacks confidence in its ability to change the lives of its members. Participation as a tool for cultural empowerment is an important health education approach that is an essential foundation for the kind of learning opportunities that empower both students/audiences and teachers/facilitators.

In order to realize fully the benefits of empowerment as a process that situates students/audiences as actors rather than factors, subjects rather than objects, and spectators rather than spectacles, cultural and educational theorists must examine and analyze the historical genealogy of classical pedagogy that disempowers the learner in a manner that Freire refers to as the "castration of curiosity" (in Freire & Faundez, 1989, p. 35). Classical pedagogy places patriarchy, White and middle-class, at the center of discourse, and at the same time maintains Others—non-Western cultures, racial and ethnic minorities, women, and low social economic classes—at the margin. Ultimately, a pedagogy of culture is needed to centralize and affirm differences in cultural expressions, thus empowering learners to be actors and subjects in the production of knowledge and their social and cultural identity. In this final chapter, I discuss the basic tenets of critical and border pedagogy, explore how this radical process informs health promotion within the context of culture, and discuss the need for health educators to promote diversity by centralizing hitherto marginalized groups in programs and curriculum development.

It has been argued that the preventive-medical model of health promotion/disease prevention efforts has a tendency to blame the victim, whereas the radical-political model may bias consciousness-raising efforts toward the interests of the health educators rather than those of the community. Under such a model, etic analysis is used when emic interpretation is not only customary but logical and empowering. In *Learning to Question* (Freire & Faundez, 1989), Freire relates an incident that took place in Mexico: An agronomist who was engaged in agricultural education through extension activities decided to help the Mexican peasants by proposing that the farmers replace their simple variety of maize with a hybrid variety to achieve greater yield in productivity. The farmers tried the hybrid successfully but subsequently changed back to their original maize variety. Had the agronomist engaged the farmers in the production and acquisition of taste, meaning, and pleasure in what was to be their new cultural reality, he would have learned, as he did later, that this simple variety of maize was grown for home consumption only and not for sale, as he had erroneously assumed. Most important, the farmers grew the simple variety of maize "to eat in their *tortillas* and the taste of the hybrid variety of maize was completely different from the other and thus represented a basic change in the culture of that community in the form of the taste of their *tortillas*" (p. 93).

Another example comes from my experience as a health education consultant for USAID in Nigeria in 1990. As part of the community's income-generating activities, the farmers were encouraged to grow their yams with fertilizers for higher yield. They tried fertilizers successfully for a year, but then discontinued their use. The yams that were grown with fertilizers rotted after two months of storage, whereas the nonfertilized yams could be stored successfully for the six months that would elapse before the planting of yams in the new season. Yet another example is the distribution of oral rehydration solution packets, as described in Chapter 6. These packets eventually create dependency instead of empowering people (Werner, 1989), who should be taught to prepare their own solution using local ingredients and implements. "The 'technical aid' conception of education 'anesthetizes' the educatees and leaves them a-critical and naive in the face of the world" (Freire, 1973, p. 152).

Empowerment in health promotion is often defined as "a process of helping people to assert control over the factors which affect their health" (Gibson, 1991, p. 369). It has also been used synonymously with such indices as coping skills, mutual support, community organization, support systems, neighborhood participation, personal efficacy, competence, self-esteem, and self-sufficiency (Kieffer, 1984; Rappaport, 1981, 1984). This concept of empowerment evokes the notion that the control of environmental forces is the ultimate goal. Although this may be true, understanding those forces in order to initiate necessary transformations of reality is a legitimate outcome of empowerment. Thus the objective changes resulting from empowerment are different because they reflect the varied needs of individuals, groups, organizations, and communities, and the contexts where empowerment occurs.

Empowerment should begin with educational institutions, so as to enlighten every student about the experiences and histories of diverse national and international communities (Airhihenbuwa & Lowe, 1994). Such institutionalization of empowerment is the hallmark of critical and border pedagogy.

## Critical Pedagogy and Culture

Paulo Freire (1970, 1973) revolutionized pedagogical approaches more than 30 years ago by bringing to the fore the debate over European-centered versus multicultural pedagogy. Classical pedagogy disempowers students and audiences by, among other things, assuming that students can only acquire knowledge, not produce it. This pedagogical approach, or what Freire (1970) refers to as "banking education," totalizes the curriculum and pedagogical practices with White, male, Western culture at the center, while marginalizing diverse student cultures and histories (Giroux, 1992). The pedagogical manifestations of this monocentric all-or-nothing discourse have been challenged in cultural studies. Grossberg (1994) offers an alternative approach to cultural studies that is a confluence of hierarchical practice, which assumes the role of the all-knowing teacher; dialogic practice, which allows the silenced to speak; and praxical pedagogical practice, which offers people the skills they need to change their destiny. Grossberg's alternative approach refuses to assume intellectual claims to authority even though the teacher does not have to abandon the position of authority.

In other words, the teacher/interventionist refuses to assume ahead of time that he or she has the appropriate knowledge, language, or skills; instead, he or she engages people in a contextual practice in which he or she is willing to risk making connections, drawing lines, mapping articulations between different domains, discourses, and practices, to see what will work, both theoretically and practically. In fact, one could relate the three approaches in cultural studies to the three approaches in health education. The hierarchical approach in cultural studies is similar to the preventive-medical approach in health education; the dialogic approach in cultural studies is similar to the radical-political approach in health education; and praxical pedagogical approach in cultural studies is similar to the empowerment model in health education. Finally, the alternative approach proposed by Grossberg is similar to the PEN-3 model I have proposed for grounding health concerns in cultural codes at both micro and macro levels of society. The connectedness between these alternative approaches is evident in the theoretical and practical symbiosis between cultural studies and health promotion.

Freire and Giroux, as well as other cultural critics and educational theorists, such as Hall and Jacques (1989), Illich (1976), Thiong'O (1986), hooks (1992), West (1993), Chinweizu (1987; Chinweizu, Jemie, & Madubuike, 1983), Minh-ha (1991), and Asante (1987), have challenged political, educational, and social systems that valorize the hegemony of White patriarchy of the Western culture while at the same time marginalizing women and people of other races and cultures. Border pedagogy and the discourse of difference must become central to pedagogical reformation (by this I mean the production of knowledge and social and cultural identity in schools, communities, and work sites as well as domestic and international) in health and education. This rethinking of health and educational intervention approaches is particularly timely given the global currents of deconstruction (rejection of universal truth) of past existential boundaries and construction of new realities based on politics of representation (inclusive of health projects that represent diverse races, ethnicities, nationalities, and genders). Given the link between cultural expressions and health behaviors (Airhihenbuwa, 1993), it is critical that health education revisit the politics of its professional location in the world.

Crossing the boundaries of educational discourse, Henry Giroux (1992) deepens and transcends the possibilities of learning opportunities by invoking the engagement of students, audiences, and teachers in the production of knowledge, meaning, pleasure, and value. His critical analysis of the politics of possibilities (which he refers to as "border pedagogy"), as they relate to education and democracy, informs a broader discourse of critical pedagogy. In his book *Border Crossings*, Giroux (1992) posits that culture is a foundation for pedagogical and political issues and thus must be central to schools' functions in the shaping of particular identities, values, and histories, by producing and legitimating specific cultural narratives and resources.

> Border pedagogy points to the need for conditions that allow students to write, speak, and listen in a language in which meaning becomes multiaccentual and dispersed and resists permanent closure. . . . border pedagogy offers the opportunity for students to engage the multiple references that constitute different cultural codes, experiences, and languages. (p. 28)

Although border crossing is advocated, it should be borne in mind that the border crosser is not a race-effacing agent. People of color cannot always assume White identity in terms of representation as Whites can assume Black identity. Therefore, crossing borders may be subject to conditions of race, gender, and nationality, to mention but three.

A disciplinary engine that has been instrumental in propelling critical pedagogy to its current theoretical and practical state is cultural studies. For cultural studies, "the question of power must always be located in a field of struggle, not as a zero sum game in which one either simply wins or loses, but, rather, as an ongoing effort to change the balance and organization of forces" (Grossberg, 1994). Thus cultural studies seek to contextualize theoretical practice by rejecting the theory known in advance of practice as well as empiricism/practice without theory. "In reality, without theory we lose ourselves in the middle of the road. But, on the other hand, without practice, we lose ourselves in the air. It is only through the contradictory, dialectical relationship of practice and theory that we can find ourselves and, if we lose ourselves sometimes, we will find ourselves again in the end" (Freire, 1993, p. 132). The connection between cultural studies and health promotion is evident in the linking of the best of practice with relevant theory such that practice becomes a form of theorizing. In the model of health education for cultural appropriateness advanced in Chapter 3 (the PEN-3 method), theorizing is manifest in practice.

## Culture and Health Promotion

Health promotion programs must problematize and reappropriate empowerment processes to centralize cultural codes and meanings in ways that address how to harness existing power, which are not always evident as new ones are being tapped. Because the classical empowerment approach in health and education suggests a focus on individual actions instead of the transformation of institutional and social forces in the environment, the onus of behavioral change still tends to rest on individuals and families. Institutional and social forces that construct the production of health, education, and politics are still largely structured in a manner that oppresses and excludes the cultural and heuristic expressions of the marginalized. As Freire (1970) notes, "One of the characteristics of oppressive cultural action which is almost never perceived by the dedicated but naive professionals who are involved is the emphasis on a focalized view of problems rather than on seeing them as dimensions of a totality" (p. 137).

In approaching the issue of oppressive cultural actions within the context of health education, I will not address the retrogressive posture of neoconservatives regarding their own educational and political project, which consistently promotes Eurocentrism as universal truth. According to Giroux (1992), "The neoconservative agenda for higher education includes a call to remake higher education an academic beachhead for defending and limiting the curriculum to a narrowly defined patriarchal, Eurocentric version of the Western tradition and return to the old transmission model of teaching" (p. 93). Moreover, "Black conservatives focus on the issue of self-respect as if it were the one key that would open all doors to Black progress. They illustrate the fallacy of trying to open all doors with one key: they wind up closing their eyes to all doors except the one the key fits" (West, 1993, p. 66). Rather, I will use critical analysis of the shortcomings of the liberal agenda to inform the future direction of health education. In the words of Giroux (1992):

> Dominant strains of liberal ideology have fashioned their antiracist discourses on a Eurocentric notion of society that subordinates the discourse of ethics and politics to the rule of the market. . . . it is precisely this assumption that prevents them [liberals] from questioning how they, as a dominant group, actually benefit from racist ideologies and social relations, even as they allegedly contest such practices. (p. 115)

Herein lies the challenge faced by health educators, particularly those of us who have been told on more than one occasion that socioeconomic status is solely responsible for the disparities in health outcomes between Caucasians and people of African descent. Such reduction of health disparities to class or social formation totally undermines the incongruence between the construction of learning opportunity in the schools and the cultural expressions of the Others, whose experiences are not central to the model of learning in the schools.

> Neither sociologists nor journalists have shown much interest in depicting poor whites as a "class." In large measure, the reason is racial. For whites, poverty tends to be viewed as atypical or accidental. Among Blacks, it comes close to being seen as a natural outgrowth of their history and culture. At times, it almost appears as if white poverty must be covered up, lest it blemish the reputation of the dominant race. (Hacker, 1992, p. 100)

Central to this debate in health promotion is the need to challenge classical pedagogy that continues to valorize the White middle-class male culture while relegating Others to the status of voyeurs. A new politics of representation must be constructed to create a space in which different voices are heard and legitimated. "The new cultural politics of difference shuns narrow particularisms, parochialisms, separatisms, just as it rejects false universalisms and homogeneous totalisms" (West, 1990, p. 34). Approaches to health education should be reformulated so that pedagogical experiences centralize and affirm the experiences of the Others, whose historical and cultural experiences have hitherto been on the margin of learning experiences. Attempts to promote cultural differences in schools and communities often manifest themselves in calls for program and/or curriculum integration, although program/curriculum reformation is a more progressive approach to centralizing diversity in the learning process. In some cases, special programs are developed to redress the grievances of the marginalized. In the United States, attempts are often made to atone for racism through measures aimed at eliminating racist institutional barriers in the marketplace and at providing compensatory programs to enhance the cultural capital and skills of African Americans, as are evident in various remedial programs in education and the workplace (Giroux, 1992).

Although the elimination of institutional barriers ought to be considered in programmatic efforts, the primary tool for exclusion often lies in the Eurocentric model of learning employed in schools. For example, in contrast to the Eurocentric model, Barbara Christian (1987) has observed that African American people have always theorized in narrative forms, "in the stories we create, in riddles and proverbs, in the play with language, since dynamic rather than fixed ideas seem more to our liking" (p. 52; quoted in Giroux, 1992, p. 131). I do not mean to assert here that all African Americans are alike in their production and acquisition of knowledge, but rather to argue for the legitimation of one valued form of cultural production found among African Americans. The differences in production and acquisition of knowledge and values of many African American children are not central to school curricula. Jacqueline Jordan Irvine (1990) writes:

> White middle-class parents and white middle-class teachers used "known-answer" questions, which solicited responses to names, shapes, and colors of objects. On the other hand, the Black children and their parents engaged in more sophisticated verbal storytelling involving the uses of metaphors and analogies. In school, Black children asked questions such as "What's that like?" or "Who's he acting like?" rather than the more middle-class attributional "What's that?" (p. 23)

Professor Asa Hilliard of Georgia State University has found that White children tend to tell stories in a "linear" fashion, whereas African American children are more apt to employ a "spiral" style, similar to learning styles found in many African cultures. When given an assignment, they frequently "skip around to several apparently irrelevant topics before they come back to the theme, and then they begin to work on it" (cited in Hacker, 1992, p. 172).

Educational reforms that focus on legitimating cultural differences have important implications for research methods. "The general method of oral history research has appeal to Black/Africana Studies because of the importance of oral communication in the historical experiences of peoples of African descent" (Stewart, 1992, p. 15). Such a focus on the significance of orature in research methods does not compromise the value of other hitherto exalted research methods; rather, it deepens and extends the possibilities for understanding cultural productions among people of African descent. African Americans, for example, must construct multivalent and multidimensional responses that articulate the complexity and diversity of their practices in the modern and postmodern world (West, 1990). If diversity is not central to the construction of learning opportunities in U.S. schools, the reality for African countries is even more troubling. The fixation on seeking so-called universal truths (the melting pot mentality) has negatively influenced the learning possibilities that legitimate and affirm different cultural meanings (the salad bowl paradigm) (Airhihenbuwa & Pineiro, 1988). The result has been the development and implementation of health programs that fail to recognize and centralize cultural influences of health practices and behavior.

## Conclusion

The future of health promotion and disease prevention strategies as components of the operationalization of health, education, and development goals lies in the ability to centralize the discourse on culture and the politics of representation at the core of programmatic and philosophical enterprise. Such a process should include the inscription of culture at the core of preventive health programs at the same time they draw on cultural studies, philosophy, education, and the traditional disciplines of influence, such as medicine and sociology, to retheorize and reconstruct health education. Grounding a health promotion episteme in the ideologies and concepts advanced in critical/border pedagogy will be a step in the right direction.

A pedagogy of culture should become central to health promotion intervention strategies in a manner that does not naturally couple the concept of barriers with cultural differences. Programmatic efforts should deepen the possibilities of critical pedagogy as a part of health promotion practices in schools, communities, and work sites, as well as at national and international levels.

# *Conclusion*

> Cultural hegemony is never about pure victory or pure domination. . . . it is never a zero sum cultural game; it is always about shifting the balance of power in the relations of culture; it is always about changing the dispositions and the configurations of cultural power, not getting out of it. There is a kind of "nothing ever changes, the system always wins" attitude, which I read as the cynical protective shell that, I am sorry to say, American cultural critics frequently wear, a shell that sometimes prevents them from developing cultural strategies that can make a difference. It is as if, in order to protect themselves against the occasional defeat, they have to pretend they can see right through everything—and it's just the same as it always was.
>
> *Stuart Hall, "What Is This 'Black' in Black Popular Culture?" 1992*

Emerging critical discourses of feminism, postmodernism, and postcolonialism have been successful in remapping the terrain of progressive theoretical discourses. These discourses have been successful neither in recognizing the importance of pedagogy as a political project (Giroux, 1994a) nor in accenting health as cultural production in the politics of representation. What I have attempted in this book is to accent culture within the context of health as one insurgent strand in these discourses. Thus it was necessary for me to challenge existing public health praxis by decentering traditional views of health, education, and development and inserting the formerly omitted element of culture into their theories and practices. No critical educator, theorist, or behavioral or social scientist can afford to ignore the relationship of health to culture and vice versa.

As I have noted in the preceding chapters, a major requirement in engaging a healthy culture project is that we move beyond the decolonization of classical paradigms and the decolonization of present Eurocentric and patriarchal professional practices. "Decolonization often means dewesternization as taught by the White man. The latter continues to arrogate the right to tell the previously colonized how to unshackle themselves, and to pronounce whether so and so has successfully returned to his or her own kind" (Minh-ha, 1991, p. 20). Decolonization is a cleansing enterprise that must be engaged by both the colonizers and the colonized. Although attempts have been made to problematize the hegemonic tools of oppression that privilege the West and patriarchy, it is equally important that the oppressed critically interrogate their position so as to expunge from their minds theories and practices that are embedded in a colonial mentality. "The decolonization of the African mind must therefore be seen as a collective enterprise, as a communal exorcism through an intellectual bath in which we need one another's help to scrub those nooks of our minds which we cannot scrub by ourselves" (Chinweizu, 1987, p. 9). Equally as important as decolonizing the minds of the marginalized is decolonizing the minds of the colonial masters. Scholarship that explores the minds, imaginations, and behaviors of the oppressed is valuable, but equally valuable is a serious intellectual effort to examine what racial ideology does to the minds, imaginations, and behaviors of oppressors (Morrison, 1992). Understanding the psychosocial functions of the role of racism in the minds of the oppressors is critical to the development and planning, for example, of cultural sensitivity workshops that should benefit the dominant population. By emphasizing the importance of the unconscious and questioning the validity of a universal subject as the center of signification, Africans are demanding a new understanding of the human sciences and a redefinition of anthropology, history, and psychoanalysis (Mudimbe, 1988).

This process challenges the oppressed to become engaged in politicizing and constructing health, education, and "development" projects for the production of knowledge and codes that are consistent with their cultural meanings. It also demands that the privileged ideology must understand and affirm the importance and "seriousness" of the scholarly projects of the Others who engage in linking the political with the practical as a theorizing enterprise. According to Derrick Bell (1992), in the United States, ethnic minority educators

> whose research is oriented toward political or practical issues are often dismissed as having introduced ideological concerns into scholarship. As a result, the selection process favors Blacks who reject or minimize their Blackness, exhibit little empathy for or interest in Black students, and express views on racial issues far removed from positions held by most Blacks including—often enough—the student groups who urge the hiring of more minority teachers. (p. 140)

Politics and education must be understood in their symbiotic roles in the production, distribution, and acquisition of knowledge. Excising the political from the life of the mind is analogous to a trembling hypochondriac always insisting on undergoing unnecessary surgery in spite of the sacrifice and high cost (Morrison, 1992). If politics is educational and education is political, outcomes should be measured by the extent to which politics and education equate culture-specific and culture-relevant health status with transformative and historical possibilities.

The affirmation of "Otherness" invoked in the politics of representation also underscores a recognition that Others are torchbearers whose political and educational projects often lead to the discovery of new truths as well as the affirmation of old truths. Quite often, when writers of oppressed races and nationalities insist that all writing is political, the claim has been dismissed as foolish or simply ignored, but when the claim is made by European philosophers it is taken up as a new and original "truth" (Alcoff, 1991-1992). On a similar plain, the unimodal analysis of Western culture for universal applications has misguided scholars into concluding that if a person's work appears similar in style and theme to previous work, he or she must have been influenced by such "Western" work. Although this may sometimes be the case, it does not hold true within the context of multiple truths.

As Chinweizu (1987) has aptly observed, because I am older than you does not mean I am your father. Such counterpoise challenges particularly the notion of role modeling that valorizes references to mostly dead White men while relegating women and colonized groups to the status of spectacles and never spectators. Consequently, it is believed that the only kinds of truths a spectacle can produce are the kinds that are good enough only for other spectacles, because original truths, which are considered the universal truths, can be produced only by spectators. Truth, like common sense, is not common or universal—it is relative and must be understood and interrogated within the politics, time, and space of particular locations.

Health promotion and disease prevention programs designed for African countries should foreground African philosophy, its cultural codes, values, and practices, in order to authenticate relevance in program outcome. This book echoes what has long been recognized—that is, any attempt to provide health solutions for a given community or society must take into serious consideration cultural factors as well as the present stage of the transformation of the society. Thus the degree to which new programs are adopted is dependent on the extent to which they are culturally appropriate. Program planners and implementers should ensure that the method of health communication is in accord with the cultural reality consistent with the society's pattern of knowledge acquisition. In order for this to occur, the health promoters must understand, learn, and develop the skills they will need to reflect appropriately the cultural values of the target population. Doing this requires an understanding not only of the cultural significance of health behaviors but also of the interplay between culture and power relative to policy formulations and decision making at the multilayered levels of a society and its government.

A major aspect of this process entails an understanding of how people promote and/or challenge policies that affect them within their cultural codes and meanings. In other words, one cannot assume that people are disempowered to make decisions based on their economically disadvantaged location. Women and other marginalized groups have always devised passive resistance strategies to subvert oppression. This point can be illustrated by the story of the wise bird. There was once a man who found a beautiful bird, fell in love with it, and decided that he wanted it for a pet. He captured the bird, brought it home, and kept it in a cage. After some days, the man asked the bird if there was anything he could do for the bird. "Of course," the bird responded, "you can open this cage." "I am sorry I cannot do that," said the man, "but I can take a message to your family to let them know that you are in good health." The bird agreed, and off the man went to find the bird's family. He successfully located the family and delivered the message of the bird's good health and safety. Upon hearing the news, one of the bird's brothers fell down dead. The man was shocked at what had happened and could not wait to get home to relate the sad event to "his" bird. Upon hearing the news about his brother, and to the man's surprise, the bird the man had imprisoned also dropped dead. The man, now filled with sorrow, opened the cage, and the bird quickly got up and flew out. As he flew away, he sang to the man, "Thank you for bringing me the wisdom of my people."

The collective experience of a people (the culture) prepares them to deal with and sometimes subvert and transform oppressive conditions in ways unknown to the oppressor. Such experiences and their resultant wisdom transcend levels of income, age, and generation. We must never assume that because a group is economically poor its members are also cerebrally, philosophically, and practically poor, nor should we assume that wisdom in and of itself will overcome economic oppression. Programmatic efforts must, therefore, be directed toward synchronizing the philosophy of the people with their practices. According to Ngugi Thiong'O (1993), what is needed is philosophy of practice rather than practical philosophy. We must transform the propagation of binary opposition between the local and the universal, particularly as it relates to culture rather than universalist dogma, which postulates that cultures within a nation and between nations have developed on parallel lines toward parallel ends that never meet.

The challenge for professionals in health and education is to learn to interrogate their relatively privileged position before adopting any strategy for improving health conditions. Empowerment of and participation by the people a program is intended to benefit must take into account the degree to which individual decisions are mediated by power, politics, class, and cultural understanding of the meaning of participation and empowerment. Empowerment must be interrogated to address the heightened sense of anxiety that may result from raising individuals' consciousness without also supplying them with the skills, power, and knowledge they need to engage the kinds of emancipatory decisions their new awareness encourages. To engage in a healthy culture project is to question one's location constantly, always remembering that when something stands, another thing always stands beside it.

# Appendix: Tables

**Table 1** Status of Women

| *African Country* | *Life Expectancy at Birth (years) 1990* | *Maternal Mortality Rate (per 100,000 live births) 1988* | *Literacy Rate (ages 15-24 only) 1980-1989* | *Women in Labor Force (% of total) 1990* |
|---|---|---|---|---|
| Algeria | 66.1 | 210 | 60 | 4 |
| Angola | 47.1 | 900 | — | 39 |
| Benin | 48.7 | 800 | 18 | 24 |
| Botswana | 62.8 | 300 | — | 35 |
| Burkina Faso | 49.9 | 750 | 7 | 49 |
| Burundi | 50.2 | 800 | — | — |
| Cameroon | 55.3 | 550 | 59 | 30 |
| Central African Republic | 52.0 | 650 | 18 | 46 |
| Chad | 48.1 | 800 | — | 17 |
| Comoro Islands | 55.5 | 500 | 55 | 41 |
| Congo | 56.3 | 900 | — | 39 |
| Côte d'Ivoire | 55.2 | 680 | — | 34 |
| Djibouti | 49.7 | 740 | — | — |
| Egypt | 61.5 | 300 | 38 | 11 |
| Equatorial Guinea | 48.6 | 800 | — | 36 |
| Ethiopia | 47.1 | 900 | — | 42 |
| Gabon | 54.2 | 600 | — | 38 |
| Gambia | 45.6 | 1,000 | — | 41 |
| Ghana | 56.8 | 700 | — | 40 |
| Guinea | 44.0 | 1,000 | — | 30 |
| Guinea-Bissau | 44.1 | 1,000 | 18 | 42 |

*(continued)*

**Table 1** Continued

| *African Country* | *Life Expectancy at Birth (years) 1990* | *Maternal Mortality Rate (per 100,000 live births) 1988* | *Literacy Rate (ages 15-24 only) 1980-1989* | *Women in Labor Force (% of total) 1990* |
|---|---|---|---|---|
| Kenya | 61.7 | 400 | — | 40 |
| Lesotho | 61.8 | 350 | — | 44 |
| Liberia | 55.5 | 600 | — | 31 |
| Madagascar | 56.0 | 600 | — | 40 |
| Malawi | 48.7 | 500 | — | 42 |
| Mali | 46.6 | 850 | 14 | 16 |
| Mauritania | 48.7 | 800 | — | 22 |
| Mauritius | 72.2 | 130 | — | 35 |
| Morocco | 63.7 | 270 | — | 20 |
| Mozambique | 49.2 | 800 | 25 | 48 |
| Namibia | 58.8 | 400 | — | 24 |
| Niger | 47.1 | 850 | — | 47 |
| Nigeria | 53.3 | 750 | — | 20 |
| Papua New Guinea | 55.7 | 700 | — | 39 |
| Rwanda | 51.2 | 700 | 45 | 48 |
| São Tomé and Príncipe | — | — | 74 | — |
| Senegal | 49.3 | 750 | — | 26 |
| Seychelles | — | — | — | 42 |
| Sierra Leone | 43.6 | 1,000 | — | 33 |
| Somalia | 47.6 | 900 | — | 39 |
| South Africa | 64.7 | 250 | — | 33 |
| Sudan | 52.0 | 700 | — | 29 |
| Swaziland | 58.6 | 400 | 75 | 40 |
| Tanzania | 55.7 | 600 | 54 | 48 |
| Togo | 55.8 | 600 | 36 | 37 |
| Tunisia | 67.5 | 200 | 63 | 13 |
| Uganda | 53.7 | 700 | — | 41 |
| Zaire | 54.7 | 700 | — | 36 |
| Zambia | 55.5 | 600 | — | 29 |
| Zimbabwe | 61.4 | 330 | — | 35 |

SOURCE: Adapted from the *Human Development Report 1993* by the United Nations Development Programme. 

**Table 2** Child Survival and Development

| *African Country* | *Low-Birth-Weight Babies (%) 1986-1990* | *Birth-Mortality Rate (per 1,000 live births) 1991* | *Children Breast-Fed at 12-15 Months (%) 1986-1991* | *1-Year-Olds Immunized (%) 1989-1991* | *Under-5 Mortality Rate (per 1,000 live births) 1990* |
|---|---|---|---|---|---|
| Algeria | — | 65 | — | 90 | 98 |
| Angola | 15 | 128 | — | 33 | 292 |
| Benin | 10 | 88 | 76 | 74 | 147 |
| Botswana | 8 | 62 | 77 | 85 | 85 |
| Burkina Faso | 12 | 120 | 97 | 50 | 228 |
| Burundi | — | 108 | 96 | 86 | 192 |
| Cameroon | 13 | 66 | — | 61 | 148 |
| Central African Republic | 18 | 106 | — | 86 | 169 |
| Chad | — | 125 | — | 33 | 216 |
| Comoro Islands | 13 | 92 | — | 94 | 151 |
| Congo | — | 83 | 90 | 81 | 110 |
| Côte d'Ivoire | 15 | 93 | 78 | 50 | 136 |
| Djibouti | 9 | 115 | — | 88 | — |
| Egypt | 12 | 59 | 77 | 87 | 85 |
| Equatorial Guinea | 10 | 120 | — | 85 | 206 |
| Ethiopia | 10 | 125 | 95 | 46 | 220 |
| Gabon | 10 | 97 | — | 82 | 164 |
| Gambia | 10 | 135 | — | 89 | 238 |
| Ghana | — | 84 | 94 | 64 | 140 |
| Guinea | 11 | 137 | 85 | 26 | 237 |
| Guinea-Bissau | 12 | 143 | 98 | 52 | 246 |
| Kenya | 15 | 68 | 83 | 71 | 108 |
| Lesotho | 10 | 82 | 76 | 81 | 129 |
| Liberia | — | 131 | 67 | 43 | 205 |
| Madagascar | 10 | 113 | 85 | 48 | 176 |
| Malawi | 11 | 144 | 96 | 84 | 253 |
| Mali | 10 | 162 | 90 | 52 | 284 |
| Mauritania | 10 | 120 | 89 | 41 | 214 |
| Mauritius | 8 | 22 | 40 | 90 | 28 |
| Morocco | 9 | 72 | 62 | 84 | 112 |
| Mozambique | 11 | 149 | — | 52 | 297 |
| Namibia | 14 | 73 | 73 | 58 | 167 |
| Niger | 20 | 127 | 15 | 24 | 221 |
| Nigeria | 17 | 99 | 86 | 66 | 167 |
| Rwanda | 16 | 112 | 74 | 86 | 198 |
| São Tomé and Príncipe | 7 | 68 | — | 71 | — |
| Senegal | 10 | 82 | 93 | 69 | 185 |
| Seychelles | 10 | 17 | — | 88 | — |

*(continued)*

**Table 2** Continued

| *African Country* | *Low-Birth-Weight Babies (%) 1986-1990* | *Birth-Mortality Rate (per 1,000 live births) 1991* | *Children Breast-Fed at 12-15 Months (%) 1986-1991* | *1-Year-Olds Immunized (%) 1989-1991* | *Under-5 Mortality Rate (per 1,000 live births) 1990* |
|---|---|---|---|---|---|
| Sierra Leone | 13 | 146 | 92 | 85 | 257 |
| Somalia | — | 125 | 54 | 24 | 215 |
| South Africa | — | 55 | — | 71 | 88 |
| Sudan | 15 | 102 | 80 | 64 | 172 |
| Swaziland | 7 | 76 | — | 90 | 167 |
| Tanzania | 16 | 104 | 70 | 86 | 170 |
| Togo | 32 | 88 | 95 | 68 | 147 |
| Tunisia | — | 45 | 57 | 92 | 62 |
| Uganda | — | 105 | 86 | 82 | 164 |
| Zaire | 10 | 96 | 86 | 40 | 130 |
| Zambia | — | 85 | 93 | 83 | 122 |
| Zimbabwe | 6 | 61 | 90 | 71 | 87 |

SOURCE: Adapted from the *Human Development Report 1993* by the United Nations Development Programme. 

**Table 3** Trends in Human Development

| African Country | Life Expectancy at Birth (years) | | Infant Mortality (per 1,000 live births) | | Population With Access to Safe Water (%) | | Daily Calorie Supply (as % of requirements) | |
|---|---|---|---|---|---|---|---|---|
| | 1960 | 1990 | 1960 | 1991 | 1975-1980 | 1988-1990 | 1965 | 1988-1990 |
| Algeria | 47.0 | 65.1 | 168 | 65 | 77 | 69 | 72 | 123 |
| Angola | 33.0 | 45.5 | 208 | 128 | 17 | 38 | 81 | 80 |
| Benin | 35.0 | 47.0 | 185 | 88 | 34 | 50 | 88 | 104 |
| Botswana | 45.5 | 59.8 | 116 | 62 | — | — | 88 | 97 |
| Burkina Faso | 36.2 | 48.2 | 205 | 120 | 25 | 67 | 91 | 94 |
| Burundi | 41.3 | 48.5 | 153 | 108 | 29 | 38 | 103 | 84 |
| Cameroon | 39.2 | 53.7 | 163 | 66 | — | — | 89 | 95 |
| Central African Republic | 38.5 | 49.5 | 175 | 106 | — | — | 91 | 82 |
| Chad | 34.8 | 46.5 | 195 | 125 | — | — | 99 | 73 |
| Comoro Islands | 42.5 | 55.0 | 165 | 92 | — | — | — | — |
| Congo | 41.6 | 53.7 | 143 | 83 | 38 | 20 | 101 | 103 |
| Côte d'Ivoire | 39.2 | 53.4 | 163 | 93 | — | — | 102 | 111 |
| Djibouti | 36.0 | 48.0 | 186 | 115 | 42 | 43 | — | — |
| Egypt | 46.1 | 60.3 | 179 | 59 | 75 | 86 | 97 | 132 |
| Equatorial Guinea | 36.8 | 47.0 | 188 | 120 | — | — | — | — |
| Ethiopia | 36.0 | 45.5 | 175 | 125 | 8 | 18 | 77 | 73 |
| Gabon | 40.8 | 52.5 | 171 | 97 | — | — | 81 | 104 |
| Gambia | 32.3 | 44.0 | 213 | 135 | — | — | — | — |
| Ghana | 45.0 | 55.0 | 132 | 84 | 35 | 56 | 87 | 93 |
| Guinea | 33.6 | 43.5 | 203 | 137 | 14 | 33 | 81 | 97 |
| Guinea-Bissau | 34.0 | 42.5 | 201 | 143 | 10 | 25 | — | — |
| Kenya | 44.7 | 59.7 | 124 | 68 | 17 | 28 | 98 | 89 |
| Lesotho | 42.9 | 57.3 | 149 | 82 | 17 | 46 | 89 | 93 |
| Liberia | 41.2 | 54.2 | 184 | 131 | — | — | 94 | 98 |
| Madagascar | 40.7 | 54.5 | 220 | 113 | — | — | 108 | 95 |
| Malawi | 37.8 | 48.1 | 207 | 144 | 51 | 53 | 91 | 88 |
| Mali | 34.8 | 45.0 | 210 | 162 | — | — | 83 | 96 |
| Mauritania | 35.3 | 47.0 | 191 | 120 | — | — | 88 | 106 |
| Mauritius | 59.1 | 69.6 | 7 | 22 | 99 | 100 | 103 | 28 |
| Morocco | 46.7 | 62.0 | 163 | 72 | — | — | 92 | 125 |
| Mozambique | 37.3 | 47.5 | 190 | 149 | — | — | 86 | 77 |
| Namibia | 42.5 | 57.5 | 146 | 73 | — | — | — | — |
| Niger | 35.3 | 45.5 | 192 | 127 | — | — | 85 | 95 |
| Nigeria | 39.5 | 51.5 | 190 | 99 | — | — | 95 | 93 |
| Rwanda | 42.3 | 49.5 | 150 | 112 | 68 | 64 | 73 | 82 |

*(continued)*

**Table 3** Continued

| *African Country* | *Life Expectancy at Birth (years)* 1960 | 1990 | *Infant Mortality (per 1,000 live births)* 1960 | 1991 | *Population With Access to Safe Water (%)* 1975-1980 | 1988-1990 | *Daily Calorie Supply (as % of requirements)* 1965 | 1988-1990 |
|---|---|---|---|---|---|---|---|---|
| São Tomé and Príncipe | — | — | — | — | — | — | — | — |
| Senegal | 37.2 | 48.3 | 172 | 82 | 36 | 53 | 104 | 98 |
| Seychelles | — | — | — | — | 79 | 99 | — | — |
| Sierra Leone | 31.5 | 42.0 | 219 | 146 | 14 | 43 | 79 | 83 |
| Somalia | 36.0 | 46.1 | 175 | 125 | 38 | 56 | 92 | 81 |
| South Africa | 49.0 | 61.7 | 89 | 55 | — | — | 107 | 128 |
| Sudan | 38.7 | 50.8 | 170 | 102 | — | — | 79 | 87 |
| Swaziland | 40.2 | 56.8 | 157 | 76 | 43 | 30 | — | — |
| Tanzania, | 40.5 | 54.0 | 147 | 104 | 39 | 52 | 85 | 95 |
| Togo | 39.3 | 54.0 | 182 | 88 | 16 | 71 | 101 | 99 |
| Tunisia | 48.3 | 66.7 | 159 | 45 | 35 | 65 | 94 | 131 |
| Uganda | 43.0 | 52.0 | 133 | 105 | 35 | 15 | 96 | 93 |
| Zaire | 41.3 | 53.0 | 158 | 96 | 19 | 34 | 98 | 96 |
| Zambia | 41.6 | 54.4 | 135 | 85 | 42 | 59 | 91 | 87 |
| Zimbabwe | 45.3 | 59.6 | 110 | 61 | — | — | 87 | 94 |

SOURCE: Adapted from the *Human Development Report 1993* by the United Nations Development Programme. Copyright © 1993. Reprinted by permission of Oxford University Press, Inc.

**Table 4** Trends in Human Development

| African Country | Adult Literacy Rate (%) 1970 | Adult Literacy Rate (%) 1990 | Combined Primary and Secondary Enrollment Ratio 1970 | Combined Primary and Secondary Enrollment Ratio 1987-1990 | Public Expenditure on Education (as % of GNP) 1988-1990 | Public Expenditure on Health (as % of GNP) 1988-1990 |
|---|---|---|---|---|---|---|
| Algeria | 25 | 57 | 46 | 79 | 9.1 | 6.0 |
| Angola | 12 | 42 | — | — | 7.3 | 1.8 |
| Benin | 16 | 23 | 23 | 37 | — | 5.1 |
| Botswana | 41 | 74 | 46 | 88 | 5.6 | 3.2 |
| Burkina Faso | 8 | 18 | 18 | 21 | 2.3 | — |
| Burundi | 20 | 50 | 18 | 39 | 3.5 | 6.0 |
| Cameroon | 33 | 54 | 50 | 65 | 3.3 | — |
| Central African Republic | 16 | 38 | 36 | 41 | 2.8 | — |
| Chad | 11 | 30 | 19 | 33 | — | — |
| Comoro Islands | — | — | 19 | 52 | 4.3 | 3.3 |
| Congo | 35 | 57 | — | — | 5.5 | 3.0 |
| Côte d'Ivoire | 18 | 54 | — | — | — | 3.0 |
| Djibouti | — | — | — | — | 2.5 | — |
| Egypt | 35 | 48 | 55 | 90 | 6.0 | 5.0 |
| Equatorial Guinea | — | — | — | — | 1.7 | — |
| Ethiopia | — | — | 11 | 28 | 4.8 | 2.0 |
| Gabon | 33 | 61 | — | — | 5.7 | 3.2 |
| Gambia | — | — | 16 | 42 | 5.2 | 1.6 |
| Ghana | 31 | 60 | 52 | 58 | 3.4 | 1.2 |
| Guinea | 14 | 24 | 24 | 24 | 1.4 | 2.0 |
| Guinea-Bissau | — | — | 29 | 38 | 2.8 | 1.3 |
| Kenya | 32 | 69 | 41 | 72 | 6.4 | 2.1 |
| Lesotho | — | — | 61 | 78 | 4.0 | 1.2 |
| Liberia | 18 | 40 | — | — | 5.7 | 3.5 |
| Madagascar | 50 | 80 | 50 | 53 | 1.9 | 0.9 |
| Malawi | — | — | 23 | 52 | 3.5 | — |
| Mali | 8 | 32 | 15 | 16 | 3.3 | 0.5 |
| Mauritania | — | — | 9 | 35 | — | 5.5 |
| Mauritius | — | — | 62 | 77 | 3.5 | 2.0 |
| Morocco | 22 | 50 | 32 | 50 | 7.4 | 3.2 |
| Mozambique | 22 | 33 | 28 | 32 | — | 1.4 |
| Namibia | — | — | — | — | — | 5.0 |
| Niger | 4 | 28 | 8 | 18 | 3.1 | 1.8 |
| Nigeria | 25 | 51 | 21 | 49 | 1.7 | — |
| Rwanda | 32 | 50 | 42 | 47 | 4.2 | 0.6 |
| São Tomé and Príncipe | — | — | — | — | 4.3 | — |

*(continued)*

**Table 4** Continued

| *African Country* | *Adult Literacy Rate (%)* | | *Combined Primary and Secondary Enrollment Ratio* | | *Public Expenditure on* | |
|---|---|---|---|---|---|---|
| | | | | | *Education (as % of GNP)* | *Health (as % of GNP)* |
| | *1970* | *1990* | *1970* | *1987-1990* | *1988-1990* | *1988-1990* |
| Senegal | 12 | 38 | 24 | 38 | — | 1.8 |
| Seychelles | — | — | — | — | 9.1 | — |
| Sierra Leone | 13 | 21 | 22 | 34 | 1.4 | — |
| Somalia | 3 | 24 | 7 | 14 | 0.4 | — |
| South Africa | — | — | — | — | — | — |
| Sudan | 17 | 27 | 24 | 36 | 4.8 | 0.3 |
| Swaziland | — | — | 63 | 85 | 7.2 | 5.8 |
| Tanzania, | — | — | 24 | 40 | 5.8 | — |
| Togo | 17 | 43 | 39 | 64 | 5.2 | 3.5 |
| Tunisia | 31 | 65 | 64 | 80 | 6.0 | 2.4 |
| Uganda | 41 | 48 | 25 | 51 | 3.4 | — |
| Zaire | 42 | 72 | — | — | 0.9 | 5.6 |
| Zambia | 52 | 73 | 61 | 67 | 2.9 | 5.1 |
| Zimbabwe | 55 | 67 | 47 | 88 | 8.2 | 5.5 |

SOURCE: Adapted from the *Human Development Report 1993* by the United Nations Development Programme. Copyright © 1993. Reprinted by permission of Oxford University Press, Inc.

# *References*

Achebe, C. (1987). *Anthills of the savannah.* Garden City, NY: Anchor/Doubleday.

Ademuwagun, Z. A. (1974-1975). The meeting point of orthodox health personnel and traditional healers/midwives in Nigeria: The pattern of utilization of health services in Ibarapa Division. *Rural Africana, 26,* 55-78.

Airhihenbuwa, C. O. (1987). Nigerian heads of households' attitude toward modern and traditional medicines. *Journal of Rural Health, 3*(11), 21-30.

Airhihenbuwa, C. O. (1989a). Health education for African Americans: A neglected task. *Health Education, 20*(5), 9-14.

Airhihenbuwa, C. O. (1989b). Perspectives on AIDS in Africa: Strategies for prevention and control. *AIDS Education and Prevention, 1,* 57-69.

Airhihenbuwa, C. O. (1990-1991). A conceptual model for culturally appropriate health education programs in developing countries. *International Quarterly of Community Health Education, 11*(1), 53-62.

Airhihenbuwa, C. O. (1992). Health promotion and disease prevention strategies for African-Americans. In R. L. Braithwaite & S. E. Taylor (Eds.), *Health issues in the Black community* (pp. 267-280). San Francisco: Jossey-Bass.

Airhihenbuwa, C. O. (1993). Health promotion for child survival in Africa: Implications for cultural appropriateness. *International Journal of Health Education, 12*(3), 10-15.

Airhihenbuwa, C. O., DiClemente, R. J., Wingood, G. M., & Lowe, A. (1992). HIV/AIDS education and prevention among African-Americans: A focus on culture. *AIDS Education and Prevention, 4,* 267-276.

Airhihenbuwa, C. O., & Lowe, A. G. (1994). Improving the health status of African-Americans: Empowerment as health education intervention. In I. L. Livingston (Ed.), *Handbook of Black American health: The mosaic of conditions, issues, policies and prospects* (pp. 387-398). Westport, CT: Greenwood Press.

Airhihenbuwa, C. O., Olsen, L. K., St. Pierre, R. W., & Wang, M. Q. (1989). Race and gender: An analysis of the granting of doctoral degrees in health education programs. *Health Education, 20*(3), 4-7.

Airhihenbuwa, C. O., & Pineiro, O. (1988). Cross-cultural health education: A pedagogical challenge. *Journal of School Health, 58,* 240-242.

Akerele, O. (1984). WHO's Traditional Medicine Programme: Progress and perspectives. *WHO Chronicle, 38*(2), 76-81.

Akerele, O. (1986). The best of both worlds. *Social Science and Medicine, 21,* 177-181.

Akinjogbin, I. A. (1990). Reflections on the Nigerian experience. In UNESCO, *Tradition and development in Africa today.* Paris: UNESCO. (Original work published 1987)

Alcoff, L. (1991-1992). The problem of speaking for others. *Cultural Critique, 17,* 5-32.

Aldous, J. (1969). Wives' employment status and lower-class men as husband-fathers: Support for the Moynihan thesis. *Journal of Marriage and the Family, 31,* 469-476.

Allen, W. (1978). The search for applicable theories of Black family life. *Journal of Marriage and the Family, 40,* 117-129.

American Public Health Association, Governing Council. (1974). *APHA Policy Statement 7424: Racism in the health care delivery system.* Washington, DC: Author.

Amos, V., & Parmar, P. (1984). Challenging imperial feminism. *Feminist Review, 17,* 7-19.

Anderson, C. A. (1966). Literacy and schooling on the development threshold: Some historic cases. In C. A. Anderson & M. Bowman (Eds.), *Education and economic development.* London: Frank Cass.

Asante, M. K. (1983). *Afrocentricity.* Trenton, NJ: African World Press.

Asante, M. K. (1987). *The Afrocentric idea.* Philadelphia: Temple University Press.

Auslander, W. F., Haire-Joshu, D., Houston, C. A., & Fisher, E. B. (1992). Community organization to reduce the risk of non-insulin-dependent diabetes among low-income African-American women. *Ethnicity and Disease, 2,* 176-184.

Baldwin, J. (1981). Notes on an Afrocentric theory of Black personality testing. *Western Journal of Black Studies, 5*(3), 172-179.

Bandura, A. (1977). Self-efficacy: Toward a unifying theory of behavioral change. *Psychological Review, 84,* 191-215.

Bannerman, R. H., Burton, J., & Wen-Chieh, C. (1983). *Traditional medicine and health care coverage: A reader for health administrators and practitioners.* Geneva: World Health Organization.

Basch, P. F. (1990). *International health.* New York: Oxford University Press.

Becker, M. H. (1986). The tyranny of health promotion. *Public Health Review, 14,* 15-25.

Bell, D. (1992). *Faces at the bottom of the well: The permanence of racism.* New York: Basic Books.

Bell, N. K. (1989). AIDS and women: Remaining ethical issues. *AIDS Education and Prevention, 1,* 22-30.

Braithwaite, R. L., & Lythcott, N. (1989). Community empowerment as a strategy for health promotion for Black and other minority populations. *Journal of the American Medical Association, 261,* 282-283.

Charatz-Litt, C. (1992). A chronicle of racism: The effects of the White medical community on Black health. *Journal of the National Medical Association, 84,* 717-725.

Chinweizu, & Jemie, O. (1987). *Decolonizing the African mind.* London: Sundoor.

Chinweizu, Jemie, O., & Madubuike, I. (1983). *Toward the decolonization of African literature: Vol. 1. African fiction and poetry and their critics.* Washington, DC: Howard University Press.

Chow, R. (1991). *Women and Chinese modernity: The politics of reading between West and East.* Minneapolis: University of Minnesota Press.

Christian, B. (1987). The race for theory. *Cultural Critique, 6,* 52.

Cochran, S. D. (1990). Women and HIV infection: Issues in prevention and behavior change. In V. M. Mays, G. W. Albee, & S. F. Schneider (Eds.), *Primary prevention of AIDS: Psychological approaches.* Newbury Park, CA: Sage.

Collison, M. N. K. (1992, September 30). Network of Black students hopes to create a new generation of civil rights leaders. *Chronicle of Higher Education,* pp. A28-A29.

Davidson, J. M. (1982). Physician participation in Medicaid: Background and issues. *Journal of Health Politics and Policy Law, 6,* 703.

Davis, A. Y. (1992). Black nationalism: The sixties and the nineties. In G. Dent (Ed.), *Black popular culture: A project by Michelle Wallace* (pp. 317-324). Seattle: Bay.

Davis, G. L., & Cross, H. J. (1979). Sexual stereotyping of Black males in inter-racial sex. *Archives of Sexual Behavior, 8,* 269-279.

Davis, J. N. P. (1959). The development of scientific medicine in the African kingdom of Bunga-kitara. *Medical History, 3*(49), 47.

Dawit, S., & Mekuria, S. (1993, December 7). The West just doesn't get it. *New York Times,* p. A27.

Dennis, R. E. (1985). Health beliefs and practices of ethnic and religious groups. In Watkins & Johnson (Eds.), *Removing cultural and ethnic barriers to health care.* Chapel Hill: University of North Carolina Press.

Desmond, S. M., Price, J. H., Hallinan, C., & Smith, D. (1989). Black and White perceptions of their weight. *Journal of School Health, 59,* 353-358.

Diop, C. A. (1991). *Civilization or barbarism: An authentic anthropology.* New York: Lawrence Hill.

Doyle, E., Smith, C. A., & Hosokawa, M. C. (1989). A process evaluation of a community-based health promotion program for a minority target population. *Health Education, 20*(5), 61-64.

Edelman, M. R. (1989). Black children in America. In J. Dewart (Ed.), *The state of Black America 1989* (pp. 63-76). New York: National Urban League.

Esteva, G. (1992). Development. In W. Sachs (Ed.), *The development dictionary: A guide to knowledge and power* (pp. 6-25). London: Zed.

Fanon, F. (1968). *The wretched of the earth.* New York: Grove.

Faseke, M. M. (1990). Oral history in Nigeria: Issues, problems, and prospects. *Oral History Review, 18*(1), 77-91.

Fingerhut, L. A., & Makuc, D. M. (1992). News from NCHS. *American Journal of Public Health, 82,* 1168-1170.

Fishbein, M., & Ajzen, I. (1975). *Belief, attitude, intention, and behavior: An introduction to theory and research.* Reading, MA: Addison-Wesley.

Fisher, J. D. (1988). Possible effects of reference group-based social influence on AIDS-risk behavior and AIDS prevention. *American Psychologist, 43,* 914-920.

Foster, E. V. (1963). *Treatment of African mental patients.* Paper presented at the Pan African Psychiatry Conference, Abeokuta, Nigeria.

Freire, P. (1970). *Pedagogy of the oppressed.* New York: Continuum.

Freire, P. (1973). *Education for critical consciousness.* New York: Continuum.

Freire, P. (1993). *Pedagogy of the city.* New York: Continuum.

Freire, P., & Faundez, A. (1989). *Learning to question.* New York: Continuum.

Fuglesang, A. (1973). *Applied communication in developing countries: Ideas and observations.* New York: Dag Hammarskjöld Foundation.

Fullilove, M., Fullilove, R. E., Haynes, K. K., & Gross, S. (1990). Black women and AIDS prevention: A view toward understanding the gender rules. *Journal of Sex Research, 27*(1), 47-64.

Gibson, C. H. (1991). A concept analysis of empowerment. *Journal of Advanced Nursing, 16*, 354-361.

Giroux, H. A. (1992). *Border crossings: Cultural workers and the politics of education*. New York: Routledge.

Giroux, H. A. (1994a). *Disturbing pleasures: Learning popular culture*. New York: Routledge.

Giroux, H. A. (1994b). Living dangerously: Identity politics and the new cultural racism. In H. A. Giroux & P. McLaren (Eds.), *Between borders: Pedagogy and the politics of cultural studies* (pp. 29-55). New York: Routledge.

Green, E. C. (1988). Can collaborative programs between biomedical and African indigenous health practitioners succeed? *Social Science and Medicine, 27*, 1125-1130.

Green, L. W., & Kreuter, M. W. (1991). *Health promotion planning: An educational and environmental approach* (2nd ed.). Palo Alto, CA: Mayfield.

Griffiths, W., & Knutson, A. L. (1960). The role of mass media in public health. *American Journal of Public Health, 50*, 515-523.

Gronemeyer, M. (1992). Helping. In W. Sachs (Ed.), *The development dictionary: A guide to knowledge and power* (pp. 53-69). London: Zed.

Grossberg, L. (1994). Introduction: Bringin' it all back home—pedagogy and cultural studies. In H. A. Giroux & P. McLaren (Eds.), *Between borders: Pedagogy and the politics of cultural studies* (pp. 1-25). New York: Routledge.

Gutierrez, L. M. (1990). Working with women of color: An empowerment perspective. *Social Work, 35*, 149-153.

Hacker, A. (1992). *Two nations: Black and White, separate, hostile, unequal*. New York: Ballantine.

Hale, C. B. (1992). A demographic profile of African Americans. In R. L. Braithwaite & S. E. Taylor (Eds.), *Health issues in the Black community* (pp. 6-19). San Francisco: Jossey-Bass.

Hall, E. T. (1977). *Beyond culture*. Garden City, NY: Anchor.

Hall, S. (1991). Ethnicity: Identity and difference. *Radical America, 23*(4), 9-20.

Hall, S. (1992). What is this "Black" in Black popular culture? In G. Dent (Ed.), *Black popular culture: A project by Michelle Wallace* (pp. 21-33). Seattle: Bay.

Hall, S., & Jacques, M. (1989). *New times: The changing face of politics in the 1990s*. London: Verso.

Hankins, C. A. (1990). Issues involving women, children, and AIDS primarily in the developed world. *Journal of Acquired Immune Deficiency Syndrome, 3*, 443-448.

Harrison, I. E. (1974). First International Symposium on Traditional Medical Therapy. *Medical Anthropology Newsletter, 6*(1), 10-13.

Harrison, I. E. (1984). *Colonialism, mealth (metropolitan health care) care systems, and traditional healers* (Occasional Paper No. 5). Urbana, IL: Association of Black Anthropologists.

Harrison, I. E., & Cosminsky, S. (1976). *Traditional medicine: Implications for ethnomedicine, ethnopharmacology, maternal and child health, mental health, and public health—an annotated bibliography of Africa, Latin America, and the Caribbean*. New York: Garland.

Harvey, W. B. (1988). Voodoo and Santeria: Traditional healing techniques in Haiti and Cuba. In C. I. Zeichner (Ed.), *Modern and traditional health care in developing societies: Conflict and cooperation.* New York: University Press of America.

Health trends: New vital statistics confirm worsening of Black health. (1992). *Ethnicity and Disease, 2,* 192-193.

Holzer, H. (1973). *Beyond medicine.* Chicago: Henry Regnery.

hooks, b. (1992). *Black looks: Race and representation.* Boston: South End.

hooks, b. (1993, September-October). Let's get real about feminism: The backlash, the myths, the movement. *Ms., 4,* 34-43.

Hornik, R. (1988). *What are we learning from the evaluation of the Communication for Child Survival project?* Philadelphia: University of Pennsylvania, Annenberg School for Communication, Center for International Health and Development Communication.

Horton, E. P., & Smith, J. C. (Eds.). (1990). *Statistical record of Black America.* Detroit: Gale Research.

Illich, I. (1976). *Medical nemesis: The expropriation of health.* New York: Pantheon.

Illich, I. (1992). Needs. In W. Sachs (Ed.), *The development dictionary: A guide to knowledge as power* (pp. 88-101). London: Zed.

International Union of Health Promotion and Education, World Health Organization, & U.S. Centers for Disease Control. (1991). *Meeting global health challenges: A position paper on health education.* Atlanta: Author.

Irvine, J. J. (1990). *Black students and school failure: Policies, practices, and prescriptions.* Westport, CT: Greenwood Press.

Jaccard, J., Turrisi, R., & Wan, C. K. (1990). Implications of behavioral decision theory and social marketing for designing social action programs. In J. Edwards, R. S. Tindale, L. Heath, & C. J. Posavac (Eds.), *Social influence processes and prevention.* New York: Plenum.

Jackson, A. M. (1983a). The Black patient and traditional psychotherapy: Implications and possible extensions. *Journal of Community Psychology, 11,* 303-307.

Jackson, A. M. (1983b). A theoretical model for the practice of psychotherapy with Black populations. *Journal of Black Psychology, 10*(1), 19-27.

Jacob, J. E. (1989). Black America, 1988: An overview. In J. Dewart (Ed.), *The state of Black America 1989* (pp. 1-7). New York: National Urban League.

Janzen, J. M. (1974-1975). Pluralistic legitimization of therapy systems in contemporary Zaire. *Rural Africana, 26,* 105-122.

Jones, J. (1982). *Bad blood: The Tuskegee syphilis experiment—a tragedy of race and medicine.* New York: Free Press.

Jordan, B. (1989). Cosmopolitan obstetrics: Some insights from the training of traditional midwives. *Social Science and Medicine, 28,* 925-944.

Justice, J. (1987). The bureaucratic context of international health: A social scientist's view. *Social Science and Medicine, 25,* 1301-1306.

Kaufman-Kurzrock, R. D. (1989). Cultural aspects of nutrition. *Topics in Clinical Nutrition, 4*(2), 1-6.

Keeling, R. (1992, April). *Taking the next steps in HIV prevention in young adults.* Paper presented at the Sixth International Conference on AIDS Education, Arlington, VA.

Kegley, C. F., & Saviers, A. N. (1983). Working with others who are not like me. *Journal of School Health, 53*(2), 81-85.

Kieffer, C. H. (1984). Citizen empowerment: A developmental perspective. In J. Rappaport, C. Swift, & R. Hess (Eds.), *Studies in empowerment: Steps toward understanding and action* (pp. 9-36). New York: Haworth.

Kisekka, M. N., & Otesanya, B. N. (1990). *Sexually transmitted disease as a gender issue: Examples from Nigeria and Uganda.* Unpublished manuscript.

Kreuter, M. W. (1992). PATCH: Its origin, basic concepts and links to contemporary public health policy. *Journal of Health Education, 23*(3), 135-139.

Kumanyika, S. K., & Golden, P. M. (1991). Cross-sectional differences in health status in U.S. racial/ethnic minority groups: Potential influence of temporal changes, disease, and life-style transitions. *Ethnicity and Disease, 1*, 50-59.

Kumanyika, S. K., Wilson, J. F., & Guilford-Davenport, M. (1993). Weight-related attitudes and behaviors of Black women. *Journal of the American Dietetic Association, 93*, 416-422.

Lamarine, R. J. (1989). First do no harm. *Health Education, 20*(4), 22-24.

Lambo, T. A. (1961). Mental health in Nigeria: Research and technical problems. *World Mental Health, 13.*

Lambo, T. A. (1978). Psychotherapy in Africa. *Human Nature, 1*(3), 32-39.

Last, M. (1986). The professionalization of African medicine: Ambiguities and definitions. In M. Last & G. L. Chavunduka (Eds.), *The professionalization of traditional medicine.* Manchester, UK: Manchester University Press/International African Institute.

Lau, R. R., Quadrel, M. J., & Hartman, K. A. (1990). Development and change of young adults' preventive health beliefs and behavior: Influence of parents and peers. *Journal of Health and Social Behavior, 31*, 240-259.

Leonard, P., & Jones, A. C. (1980). Theoretical considerations for psychotherapy with Black clients. In R. C. Jones (Ed.), *Black psychology* (2nd ed.). New York: Harper & Row.

Levy, D. R. (1985). White doctors and Black patients: Influence of race on the doctor-patient relationship. *Pediatrics, 75*, 639-643.

Lewin, K. (1947). Group decision and social change. In A. Swanson, T. M. Newcomb, & Z. L. Hartley (Eds.), *Readings in social psychology* (pp. 197-211). Englewood Cliffs, NJ: Prentice Hall.

Maclean, L. M., & Bannerman, R. H. (1982). Utilization of indigenous healers in national health delivery systems. *Social Science and Medicine, 16*, 1815-1816.

Malinowski, B. (1954). The rationalization of anthropology and administration. *Africa, 3*, 405-429.

Marable, M. (1993). Beyond racial identity politics: Towards a liberation theory for multicultural democracy. *Race and Class, 35*(1), 113-130.

Mariani, P., & Crary, J. (1990). In the shadow of the West: An interview with Edward Said. In R. Ferguson, W. Olander, M. Turker, & K. Fiss (Eds.), *Discourses: Conversations in postmodern art and culture.* New York/Cambridge: New York Museum of Contemporary Art/MIT Press.

Mays, V. M., & Cochran, S. D. (1988). Issues in the perception of AIDS risk and risk reduction activities by Black and Latino women. *American Psychologist, 43*, 949-957.

Mazrui, A. A. (1986). *The Africans: A triple heritage.* Boston: Little, Brown.

McNair-Knox, F. C. (1991). Tapping into teen talk: Parenting strategies for bridging the intergenerational communication gap. In B. P. Bowser (Ed.), *Black male adolescents: Parenting and education in community context*. New York: University Press of America.

McNamara, R. S. (1973, September 24). Address to the Board of Governors, World Bank, Nairobi.

Miles, G. B., & McDavis, R. J. (1982). Effects of four orientation approaches on disadvantaged Black freshmen students' attitudes toward the counseling center. *Journal of College Student Personnel, 23*, 413-418.

Minh-ha, T. T. (1989). *Woman, nature, other: Writing postcoloniality and feminism*. Bloomington: Indiana University Press.

Minh-ha, T. T. (1991). *When the moon waxes red: Representation, gender and cultural politics*. New York: Routledge.

Mitchell, J. L. (1988). Women, AIDS, and public policy. *AIDS and Public Policy Journal, 3*(2), 50-52.

Mohanty, C. T. (1991a). Introduction: Cartographies of struggle. In C. T. Mohanty, A. Russo, & L. Torres (Eds.), *Third World women and the politics of feminism* (pp. 1-47). Bloomington: Indiana University Press.

Mohanty, C. T. (1991b). Under Western eyes: Feminist scholarship and colonial discourses. In C. T. Mohanty, A. Russo, & L. Torres (Eds.), *Third World women and the politics of feminism* (pp. 51-80). Bloomington: Indiana University Press.

Morales, E. S. (1987). AIDS and ethnic minority research. *Multicultural Inquiry and Research on AIDS, 1*, 2.

Morrison, T. (1992). *Playing in the dark: Whiteness and the literary imagination*. New York: Vintage.

Mudimbe, V. Y. (1988). *The invention of Africa: Gnosis, philosophy, and the order of knowledge*. Bloomington: Indiana University Press.

Mullen, P. D., Hersey, J. C., & Iverson, D. C. (1987). Health models compared. *Social Science and Medicine, 24*, 973-981.

Muller, C. (1985). A window on the past: The position of the client in twentieth century public health thought and practice. *American Journal of Public Health, 75*, 470-476.

Myers, H. F., & King, L. M. (1983). Mental health issues in the development of the Black American child. In G. J. Powell (Ed.), *The psychosocial development of minority group children*. New York: Brunner/Mazel.

Nathanson, C. A., & Becker, M. H. (1986). Family and peer influence on obtaining a method of contraception. *Journal of Marriage and the Family, 48*, 513-525.

Newman, A., & Bhatia, J. C. (1973). Family planning and indigenous medicine practitioners. *Social Science and Medicine, 14A*, 23-29.

Nichols, M. (1990). Women and acquired immunodeficiency syndrome: Issues for prevention. In B. Voeller, J. M. Reinisch, & M. Gottlieb (Eds.), *AIDS and sex: An integrated biomedical and biobehavioral approach*. New York: Oxford University Press.

Njoku, J. E. E. (1980). *The world of the African woman*. Metuchen, NJ: Scarecrow.

Nobles, W. W. (1980). African philosophy: Foundations for Black psychology. In R. L. Jones (Ed.), *Black psychology* (2nd ed.). New York: Harper & Row.

Nobles, W. W. (1985). Back to the roots: African culture as a basis for understanding black families. In W. W. Nobles (Ed.), *Africanity and the Black family: The development of a theoretical model*. Berkeley, CA: Institute for the Advanced Study of Black Family Life and Culture.

Osuntokun, B. O. (1975). The traditional basis of neuropsychiatric practice among the Yorubas of Nigeria. *Tropical Geographic Medicine, 27,* 422-430.

Oyebola, D. D. O. (1986). National medical policies in Nigeria. In M. Last & G. L. Chavunduka (Eds.), *The professionalization of traditional medicine.* Manchester, UK: Manchester University Press/International African Institute.

Ozer, E. M., & Bandura, A. (1990). Mechanisms governing empowerment effects: A self-efficacy analysis. *Journal of Personality and Social Psychology, 58,* 472-486.

Parham, T. A., & Helms, J. E. (1985). Relation of racial identity attitudes to self-actualization and affective states of Black students. *Journal of Counseling Psychology, 32,* 431-440.

Parker, S., & Kleiner, R. (1969). Social psychological dimensions of the family role performance of the Negro male. *Journal of Marriage and the Family, 33,* 500-506.

Pedersen, P., Draguns, J., Conner, W., & Trimble, J. (1981). *Counseling across cultures.* Honolulu: University of Hawaii Press/East-West Center.

Pernick, M. S. (1985). *A calculus of suffering.* New York: Columbia University Press.

Petersdorf, P. G., Turner, K. S., Nickens, H. W., & Ready, T. (1990). Minorities and medicine: Past, present, and future. *Academic Medicine, 65,* 663-670.

Peterson, J. L., & Bakerman, R. (1989). AIDS and IV drug use among ethnic minorities. *Journal of Drug Issues, 19*(1), 27-37.

Pike, K. L. (1954). *Language in relation to a unified theory of the structure of human behavior: Part 1* (preliminary ed.). Summer Institute of Linguistics.

Pillsbury, B. L. K. (1982). Policy and evaluation perspectives on traditional health practitioners in national health care systems. *Social Science and Medicine, 16,* 1825-1834.

Proctor, E., & Rosen, A. (1981). Expectations and preferences for counselor race and their relation to intermediate treatment outcomes. *Journal of Counseling Psychology, 28,* 40-46.

Radcliffe-Brown, A. R. (1952). *Structure and function in primitive society: Essays and addresses.* Glencoe, IL: Free Press.

Rahnema, M. (1992). Participation. In W. Sachs (Ed.), *The development dictionary: A guide to knowledge and power* (pp. 116-131). London: Zed.

Rappaport, J. (1981). In praise of paradox: A social policy of empowerment over prevention. *American Journal of Community Psychology, 9,* 1-25.

Rappaport, J. (1984). Studies in empowerment: Introduction to the issue. In J. Rappaport, C. Swift, & R. Hess (Eds.), *Studies in empowerment: Steps toward understanding and action* (pp. 1-7). New York: Haworth.

Rosenstock, I. M. (1974). Historical origins of the health belief model. *Health Education Monographs, 2,* 328-335.

Sachs, W. (1992). Introduction. In W. Sachs (Ed.), *The development dictionary: A guide to knowledge and power* (pp. 1-5). London: Zed.

Saegert, S. (1989). Unlikely leaders, extreme circumstances: Older Black women building community households. *American Journal of Community Psychology, 17,* 295-316.

Savitt, T. L. (1982). The use of Blacks for medical experimentation and demonstration in the Old South. *Journal of Southern History, 48,* 331-335.

Schram, R. (1971). *A history of Nigerian health services.* Ibadan, Nigeria: Ibadan University Press.

Seidel, G. (1993). The competing discourses of HIV/AIDS in sub-Saharan Africa: Discourses of rights and empowerment vs. discourses of control and exclusion. *Social Science and Medicine, 36,* 175-194.

Seijas, H. (1975). An approach to the study of medical aspects of culture. *Current Anthropology, 14,* 344-345.

Simons, M. (1989, May 16). Poor nations seeking rewards for contributions to plant species. *New York Times,* p. 18.

Sprafka, J. M., Burke, G. L., Folsom, A. R., & Hahn, L. P. (1989). Hypercholesteremia prevalence, awareness and treatment in Blacks and Whites: The Minnesota Heart Survey. *Preventive Medicine, 18,* 423-432.

Stewart, J. B. (1989). *The state of Black studies: Perspectives from the first NCBS Summer Faculty Institute and implications of the NRC report "A common destiny."* Paper presented at Temple University, Philadelphia.

Stewart, J. B. (1992). Reaching for higher ground: Toward an understanding of Black/Africana studies. *Afrocentric Scholar, 1*(1), 1-63.

Street, B. V. (1984). *Literacy in theory and practice.* Cambridge, UK: Cambridge University Press.

Sullivan, L. W. (1989). Shattuck lecture: The health care priorities of the Bush administration. *New England Journal of Medicine, 321,* 125-128.

Teller, A. (1968). Studies on aspects of traditional medicine. *Lagos Notes and Records,* 2(1), 18.

Thiam, A. (1986). *Speak out, Black sisters: Feminism and oppression in Black Africa.* London: Pluto.

Thiong'O, N. W. (1986). *Decolonizing the mind: The politics of language in African literature.* London: James Currey/Heinemann.

Thiong'O, N. W. (1993). *Moving the center: The struggle for cultural freedoms.* London: James Currey.

Tones, K., Tilford, S., & Robinson, Y. K. (1991). *Health education: Effectiveness and efficiency.* London: Chapman & Hall.

Torrey, E. F. (1972). What Western psychotherapists can learn from witch doctors. *American Journal of Orthopsychiatry, 42,* 69-76.

U.N. Development Programme. (1993). *Human development report.* New York: Oxford University Press.

U.S. Department of Health and Human Services. (1985). *Report of the Secretary's Task Force on Black and Minority Health* (Vol. 1, exec. summary). Washington, DC: Government Printing Office.

U.S. Department of Health and Human Services. (1991). *Health of the United States and prevention profile* (NCHS Publication No. PHS 91-1232). Washington, DC: Government Printing Office.

U.S. Surgeon General. (1979). *Healthy people: The surgeon general's report on health promotion and disease prevention.* Washington, DC: Government Printing Office.

Werner, D. (1989, June 18-21). *Health for no one by the year 2000: The high cost of placing "national security" before global justice.* Address presented to the 16th Annual International Health Conference of the National Council for International Health, Arlington, VA.

West, C. (1990). The new cultural politics of difference. In R. Ferguson, M. Geverr, T. T. Minh-ha, & C. West (Eds.), *Out there: Marginalization and contemporary cultures* (pp. 19-36). Cambridge: MIT Press.

West, C. (1993). *Race matters.* Boston: Beacon.

Whitehead, T. (1992). In search of soul food and meaning: Culture, food, and health. In H. A. Baer & Y. Jones (Eds.), *African Americans in the South: Issues of race, class, and gender* (pp. 94-110, 161-178). Athens: University of Georgia Press.

World Health Organization. (1989). Memoranda: In vitro screening of traditional medicines for anti-HIV activity: Memorandum for a WHO meeting. *Bulletin of the World Health Organization, 67*, 613-618.

Wyatt, G. E., Strayer, R. G., & Lobitz, W. C. (1976). Issues in the treatment of sexual dysfunctioning couples of Afro-American descent. *Psychotherapy, 13*, 44-50.

# *Index*

# *About the Author*

**Collins O. Airhihenbuwa** is Associate Professor and Head of the Department of Health Education at the Pennsylvania State University. He earned his bachelor's degree in health care administration and planning from Tennessee State University/Meharry Medical College in Nashville, Tennessee, and his M.P.H. and Ph.D. degrees, in health care planning and administration and public health education, respectively, from the University of Tennessee in Knoxville. He has written extensively on cultural influences on health beliefs and behavior, and he has developed a culturally sensitive programmatic model for planning, implementing, and evaluating health promotion programs in Africa and other Southern regions as well as among African Americans and other ethnic minorities in the United States. On the basis of his international and cultural health research, he has been invited to lecture at the local, national, and international levels using his model as a framework. He is a consultant to several national and international agencies, including the U.S. Agency for International Development, the U.N. Development Programme, and the World Health Organization.